Secrets in Psychotherapy

This book brings together contemporary perspectives from psychodynamic treatment, advances in cognitive science, medicine, and neuroscience in a user-friendly format. guiding practitioners from beginner to more advanced levels in working with secrets that emerge during psychotherapy.

Despite their ubiquity in life and in clinical practice, secrets and secret keeping receive limited attention in the training and skill set required for mental health clinicians. Drawing on personal experience and clinical expertise, as well as film, memoir, and literature, Dr. Kathryn Zerbe shares how secrets come to light in both life and treatment, demonstrating the powerful hold that secrets can have on our lives. This book offers a fresh take on how we view our secrets and how we can use them as a tool to sustain our most intimate and valued connections over the course of a lifetime. Using cutting-edge research as well as honed clinical expertise, the author suggests how one might go about managing the secrets of everyday living that we must keep as well as how we can identify which we can let go. Particular attention is paid to the mind/body relationship and somatic countertransference reactions. Each chapter suggests guidelines to promote wellness and resilience in the secret keeper, whether they are the psychotherapist or their patient.

Written with compassion and in a user-friendly style, *Secrets in Psychotherapy* will benefit anyone who is navigating the thorny terrain of keeping a secret for themselves or someone they know. It is an essential read for psychotherapists, psychoanalysts, and practicing mental health professionals of all disciplines.

Kathryn Zerbe, MD, FABP, is a Training and Supervising Analyst, Oregon Psychoanalytic Center, and Clinical Professor of Psychiatry, Oregon Health and Sciences University. She practices in Portland, OR.

Secrets in Psychotherapy
Stories that Inform Clinical Work

Kathryn Zerbe

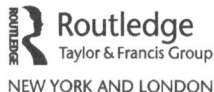
Routledge
Taylor & Francis Group

NEW YORK AND LONDON

Designed cover image: Getty Images

First published 2025
by Routledge
605 Third Avenue, New York, NY 10158

and by Routledge
4 Park Square, Milton Park, Abingdon, Oxon, OX14 4RN

Routledge is an imprint of the Taylor & Francis Group, an informa business

ISBN: 978-1-032-74930-3 (hbk)
ISBN: 978-1-032-74923-5 (pbk)
ISBN: 978-1-003-47157-8 (ebk)

DOI: 10.4324/9781003471578

Typeset in Sabon
by codeMantra

For Marshall
  and all the others
  who taught me that sharing a secret can be life saving

Contents

Acknowledgments   *xi*

Introduction   1

1 The Power of Secrets   11

2 The Burden of Secrecy   33

3 The Afterlife of a Double Life   60

4 Discovering Phantoms and Ghosts   78

5 Somatic Countertransference   101

6 The Complicated Ethics of Concealment   125

7 Hidden Talents and Abilities   149

Epilogue   168

References   *173*
Index   *189*

Acknowledgments

Years ago, a maxim from the Talmud was printed in the weekly patient newsletter at the Menninger Clinic in Topeka, Kansas: "Every blade of grass has its angel that bends over it and whispers, 'Grow, grow.'" I cut and taped it into my desk drawer. I'm thankful for the anonymous editor who had the prescience to include the passage among all the announcements of upcoming events and activities. It's a reminder that defies religious or philosophical traditions. A therapist aspires to be an earthly force for the growth of others, but she must bow to the whispering sprites she encounters who support her own need for ongoing development. I have been blessed with many over the course of my life and in every step of the way during the writing of this book.

My partner Kelli Holloway is such a force. As my first-line editor, she read multiple drafts of each chapter and helped me refine ideas and concepts as they emerged. Writing a book is work, she frequently reminded me. Astutely, she urged me to carve out slices of time in my practice and put up with seemingly endless disappearances into the "notorious black hole" of the present study over evenings and weekends. Without her gentle—and repeated—pushing, I would never have undertaken an entire writing program at this stage of life.

Some of the clinical examples and dialogue segments in this book found initial breath at New Directions in Writing, under the auspices of the Washington Baltimore Center for Psychoanalysis. During the three-year postgraduate course, I encountered gifted teachers, speakers, and other students who had much to share and supported my discovery of a voice different from the one I used in professional papers and previous books. It was a surprise to see what spontaneously percolated from free-write exercises and 750-word essay assignments that were then refined over long weekends of small group practice sessions. I am grateful to all the faculty members, seminar leaders, and other students whom I met at New Directions and who were part of this wonderful learning environment. In particular, Valerie Frankfeldt and Debra Neumann brought finely tuned clinical ears, key insights, and dollops of humor to early chapters.

At New Directions, I became reacquainted with Elizabeth McKamy, a dear friend and colleague from the Menninger years. A social worker by profession and writing instructor and seminar leader in the program, Liz grasped early on that the topic of secrets excited me as a scholarly pursuit. She had the foresight to propose that some of my ideas could be further shaped and perhaps turned into a career capstone. In time, I asked Liz to become my formal writing consultant, and she brought all her clinical acumen, authorial expertise, and probing intellect to the task, offering perceptive advice for content revision, streamlined dialogues, and clarity of prose. Liz was the essential midwife this book needed.

Kate Murphy believed in the project from its inception and encouraged me to keep going when publishers were less than enthusiastic about the topic. Carlene Benson, Paul Hamilton, and John Williams also urged me not to give up when I hit inevitable rough patches. They carefully read and reread portions of the book and offered constructive commentary as it developed. I am fortunate to have each one in my corner.

My deepest gratitude goes to the patients, supervisees, and interviewees who entrusted me with their stories and, in the process, taught me much about life. They showed me the fortitude it takes to squarely face one's truth and, no matter the scale of prior difficulty or current cost, decide to make necessary but difficult changes. Rest assured, all secrets remain safe. I've taken care to thoroughly disguise all clinical and interview material, adopt pseudonyms, and, in a few instances, make use of case composites. Everyone's story is unique, but the quicksand of secret keeping surfaces in similar territories. Readers whom I will never meet will likely not be surprised to discover elements of identification with some of the situations described in these pages.

It has been a privilege to work with outstanding editors. Without the encouragement, collaboration, and kindness of Julia Giordano, this book might not have seen the light of day or been half as rewarding to write. I am grateful for her enthusiastic support, skillfulness, and bedrock professionalism. I also wish to thank the entire production team at Routledge—Julia Giordano, Pragati Sharma, and Alice Maher—for manuscript preparation, editorial suggestions, and attention to detail. Katie Van Heest of Tweed Editing provided exquisite copyediting along with incisive comments and judicious advice that significantly improved the final version of the text.

Family continues to be an abiding source of inspiration and sustenance that enriches my world and grounds my clinical practice. Beth and Dale Holloway were the second set of parents everyone hopes to find in adult life; their love, warmth, and wisdom knew no bounds. To my great benefit, their spark lives on within Kelli.

Introduction

Introduction

When I say that secrets perplex even the sharpest clinical minds, it may come across as exaggeration. But consider the accomplished internist Dr. James and the hidden truth that became an unsuspected poison to his own family.

All the way from the back of the auditorium, Dr. James strode to the podium as the other speakers on the panel took some final questions. He bent down and whispered into my ear, "I want to talk with you after the meeting. Do you have a moment?"

I nodded. It wouldn't be polite to ignore the conference organizer who had invited me, a relatively junior clinician, to lecture at this regional internal medicine meeting on addictions in women's mental health. I suspected that he was going to offer some off-the-cuff criticism of my earlier presentation. Even if Dr. James's remarks would be well intended, I readied myself for reproof. My career as a writer and speaker in psychiatry was just getting started. I wanted to come across as unassuming and easy to work with, so the planners might invite me in the future. The advice of a respected physician would no doubt improve my performance.

"It's going to take more than a minute," Dr. James confessed later. We were crossing over the domed bridge on our way to the benches on the outdoor patio. As I tried to keep up with his quick pace, he asked, "May I buy you something to drink or a snack? Somewhere that's a little more comfortable and private?"

"Sure," I replied, then deflected to foil what I suspected might be a subtle but flattering flirtation. "But it needs to be here at the hotel because I'm catching a ride to the airport with a colleague in a couple of hours."

The deflection wasn't necessary, as it turned out. Dr. James really did want to talk. My assumption that he would begin by lighting into me was not too far off the mark, however.

"I listened to every word you said," he began. "I'm sure that the psychodynamic approach and psychological treatments you recommended are

DOI: 10.4324/9781003471578

relevant for the patients you work with, but not to me or my practice."
I encouraged him to elaborate. After continuing for just a little while, he
suddenly became crestfallen and shaky. He blanched, shrugged his shoulders, and stopped making eye contact. I sensed a turning point in our
conversation.

> Look—what I really need to talk to you about is not your speech. It's
> about my daughter. She's only nineteen and has an eating disorder.
> She exercises constantly and occasionally runs off and gets bleary eyed
> drunk. She's landed herself in with a pretty rough crowd. Her mother
> and I are worried sick about her. She refuses to go back to college or get
> a job. We've spent thousands of dollars on the treatments that you and
> the others advocated at the conference this weekend, and we don't see
> anything doing one lick of good. I am so bent out of shape. She's been a
> much tougher child to raise than her older brother and sister.

I was getting the picture. What had begun as a benign proposition for a brief
chat or curbside consultation over a sandwich turned itself into a detailed
account of not only Dr. James's daughter's problems but his own personal
history with addiction, dissatisfaction with his medical practice, and lingering resentment from his wife about his travel and work commitments.

The clock was ticking. When I attempted to steer the course of our conversation by summing things up, he shut me down. More details poured
out. I tried to signal the time by glancing at my watch. He didn't notice
and continued to spill.

> My wife doesn't appreciate that staying busy is what keeps me sane! My
> recovery program touted the benefits of maintaining a tight structure.
> Do you agree? I don't think I mentioned how my treatment wiped out
> my retirement. It nearly led to total bankruptcy! It's shameful. My colleagues treat me like a pariah.

Still relatively unseasoned to the circumlocutions that denial and resistance
use to thwart meaningful dialogue between two adults, I listened until my
brain sputtered and my body ached. "I have to catch my ride." I rose from
the booth, defeated, and grabbed my purse after nearly two hours. "I wish
the best for all of you."

"Before you go," he mustered,

> There is just one more thing that I have to tell you. Our daughter is
> adopted. Hannah doesn't know it. We've never spoken about it. You
> don't think that that has anything to do with any of her psychiatric difficulties, do you?

A secret is divulged. But precisely whose secret is it, and how might its repercussions be influencing Dr. James's family, if at all? At this moment we cannot be certain whether the consciously withheld information has any role whatsoever to play in his daughter's suffering. It's easy for anyone, especially a mental health professional, to jump to conclusions because we want to be helpful, to put some emotional salve on an open psychological wound that is obviously stirring conflict and heartache. Working with secrets, however, demands a different approach: sticking with our discomfort and nudging the distressed individual to provide a bit more detail or context.

Meeting Dr. James changed my life. The psychotherapist's privileged position affords the opportunity to follow the lead when a person confides and to always consider what may lie beneath the surface, but after my conversation with Dr. James, I began to listen for secrets and attune to them more explicitly in my clinical practice. I regret that I had relatively little to offer my colleague in the moment. I would conclude my conversation with Dr. James differently now than I did over four decades ago. In many ways, this book holds some answers that I wish that I could have provided in that poignant moment of farewell.

How might it have gone better? I vaguely recall saying something akin to how important it was to be transparent with Hannah's treatment team about the circumstances of her birth and for him to have a safe place (e.g., individual psychotherapy, group counseling) to consider the question he had just posed to me. While that was a start, now I would add that while he had valid *reasons* for this paramount decision not to reveal the fact of adoption that needed to be understood over time, any unforeseen impact on his daughter was equally important. I had neither the time nor the therapeutic contract to follow up with Dr. James, but it's clear that he carried a significant psychological burden and a wealth of associations that likely were linked together.

It's equally possible that he was not the only member of his family similarly caught in between. Let's assume that the reason that Hannah's adoption was not openly discussed in this family was a desire for her protection. While Dr. James genuinely believed that his daughter was unaware of the circumstances of her birth, I found myself wondering whether her mother or even one of her older siblings might have let the fact slip out because it was simply too hard to bury forever. Whoever might have revealed the secret then might have attempted to alleviate their guilt or anxiety by asking for Hannah's promise to never say a word about it lest Dr. James become angry, fall into depression, or start drinking again.

Tendrils of curiosity and empathy begin to extend to every member of this household as we consider their plight. Hannah James may herself be holding secrets inside. She may be disturbed because she figured out that she is adopted but got the message she cannot mention it. She may experience herself as different from others or emotionally confused but finds it nearly impossible to convey this forthrightly. Hannah's eating disorder, binge drinking, and acting out may be ways she indirectly speaks to unconscious pain related to her secrets, the bodily and psychological signals of cloudy thinking and affect intolerance brought about by layers of complicity—all undertaken with the best of intentions by those in her circle. It will take time and building trust for Hannah to be open with what she senses or feels about herself.

Sometimes, speaking openly about emotionally charged issues can be perceived as hurtful or disruptive. Were insidious messages to that effect conveyed between members of Dr. James's household? Neuroscientists now suspect that human beings expend considerable energy trying to block out what we are unable to process or fully experience. Brain-based mechanisms along what is termed the "conscious–unconscious continuum" are being studied for the key role they play in sparking and sustaining emotional dysregulation and cognitive difficulties (Ginot, 2009, 2015). These neurophysiological processes add to our understanding of the impact of keeping secrets, such as in Hannah's case.

It's common for someone to confide an intimate detail and then slam the door shut and never say another word about it again. Many clinical examples throughout this book attest to that pattern. This frequently happens in life, not just in psychotherapy, but I learned to encourage my psychotherapy supervisees and students especially to take the difficult step of going slowly with an individual who shares a confidence. The job is to keep the door propped slightly ajar by bringing an attitude of gentleness and curiosity to the conversation, so that both therapist and patient can take the next peek into the emotional storage cabinet only after the ground is well prepared. The requisite foundation of safety and empathy can be established only over time.

Another reason to engage with degrees of humility and inscrutability is that secrets are inherently complex and ambiguous communications. As the examples in this book will make abundantly clear (and that each of us intuits quite well through our life experiences), when someone tests our understanding by bursting forth with a comment, such as "There's just one more thing I need to tell you," a portal opens, and you are likely to get more of an earful than anticipated. Throughout the chapters, we will explore ways to help patients handle these kinds of revelations in family, personal, and social situations and to distinguish these circumstances from the complementary but decidedly different expectations necessary when one engages in contracted clinical work with a psychotherapist or psychoanalyst.

In the psychotherapy process, a spool of information begins to unwind that can and often does lead anywhere and everywhere and frequently gets temporarily tied in knots. The boundaries between privacy, secrecy, gossip, and outright lying are as essential to distinguish in psychotherapy as they are outside the consultation room. The distinctions can get murky and create consternation among well-meaning individuals. Listening to secrets can be and often is alleviating for the sharer, but one must always bear in mind potential unsuspected land mines that are frequently right around the corner.

In clinical practice, secrets tend to group themselves along certain themes. As we will see, the most common tend to center around these subjects:

1 Sexuality: adultery, sexual assault, discovery of an unknown half-sibling or "second, hidden" family of a parent, leading a "double life."
2 Grief and loss: miscarriage, infertility, abortion, illness, revelations after the death of a loved one.
3 Addictions: alcoholism, drugs, eating disorders, gambling, compulsive sexual behavior.
4 Death and trauma: suicide, murder, abuse, complicated bereavement, history of genocide or slavery, transgenerational transmission of trauma.
5 Money and finances: bankruptcy, embezzlement, hidden assets, wealth or poverty.
6 Criminal behavior and incarceration: ongoing acts or past misconduct of the individual or a loved one.

What is particularly fascinating is why or when concealment begins as a nidus considered trivial or innocuous by most people and gradually grows, morphs, and ultimately damages the psyche. The linchpin often rests in the perception by the individual that what has transpired is so humiliating, mortifying, or sullying as to be considered unspeakable.

Secret keeping affects mind and body. Sometimes, we try to forget what we know. The weight of what is split off from awareness that factors into psychological distress and physical illness has been surmised since the origins of psychoanalysis in the late 1800s, but now science is providing additional data about how, what, where, and when such sealed-off information may become harmful. How do we keep in mind personal facts about others that they do not want exposed but that, at the same time, may implicate us in a conspiracy of silence?

This perplexity creates in individuals what I call in my practice facts that are *hiding but in plain view*. They occur in families, intimate relationships, and friendships. I have found that the obvious is perceived as too dangerous, shameful, or potentially disruptive to openly give voice to. But it finds expression in eating disorders, addictions, depression and anxiety disorders, and attention-based learning problems. On an emotional level, a person *knows* a secret or set of secrets that they believe they *should not know*, and certainly not talk about openly. While able to stave off awareness to a certain extent by deploying the mind's elaborate defensive systems, the secret inevitably leaks out, commonly through the byway of the presenting problem or symptom that brings the individual into treatment.

This book includes patient examples of the impact of harboring what is hiding in plain sight (that is, a secret) that I have witnessed in my practice over the years. I go on to describe some of the psychotherapeutic gains made as the issues were constructively but arduously worked through over time. Chapters 1, 2, and 3 drive home aspects of the power inherent in secrecy but also its untoward physical and emotional consequences on individuals, particularly those who lead double lives or are placed in the position of guarding the secrets of loved ones.

Novels, films, memoir, and biographies are flush with situations in which we find out that a particular character is aware of secrets in their history. The plot makes a salubrious turn when this information is finally clarified, and the story concludes straightforwardly for the good of all. In real life, the mysterious human heart takes us on a far more convoluted journey. Psychoanalysis is in part the study of the impact of how many events in a person's history are warded off by denial, repression, or dissociation that serve protective functions. In therapy, a secret often comes to light after discussion of the consciously known event, an unconsciously suppressed idea, or a dissociated trauma. Psychotherapists observe that the individual often then goes to new and unpredictable lengths to ward off the impact of that new knowledge!

Why would this be the case? Since the late 1960s, and continuing right up to the present, psychoanalysts have explored the generational transmission of conflict and trauma and its impact on child development. Certain children are blocked or inhibited from normal self-expression and individuation because they are tasked with keeping a shameful or disturbing event of their parent's or grandparent's life to themselves. They are not consciously aware of this event but mysteriously enact it through their psychiatric symptoms. One question that I consider when I treat individuals today, for example, is the aftermath of some unbearable family sadness or horrific historical event that is repeated in the present and thus implicated in the range of the individual's ongoing psychological struggles. I expand on this crucial aspect of silencing throughout the book, but especially in Chapters 2 and 4.

Historical tragedies such as slavery, genocide, the Holocaust, and apartheid, as well as cultural phenomena such as cult membership or religious zealotry, are also breeding grounds for emotionally unformulated experiences that take up residence in the body or mind of the sufferer. As such, they are ready depositories for secret keeping. Relief comes in the form of finding healthy ways to give these horrific and heretofore untethered events a voice. Psychodynamic psychotherapy, or psychoanalysis, is one of those ways.

As a physician who has always been fascinated by the mind-body connection in practice, I find new data from neuroscience and cognitive psychology highly relevant to my work with patients and students in mental health, psychotherapy, and psychoanalysis. Throughout the book, I speak about some of this research and how it can be applied to understanding and helping human beings. The findings have significant implications for anyone charged with keeping secrets, be it within our professional or personal relationships. In Chapters 5 and 6, I address ways in which the body reacts or attunes to secret keeping (i.e., the clinician's somatic or embodied countertransference reactions) and the complicated ethical decision-making process thrust upon those in the secret-keeping professions. As we will see, the role not only requires ongoing self-reflection about our value system and personal boundaries but may also have unsuspected and often grave impact on the mind and body.

A secret can be a powerful piece of information; revealing it often disrupts a complicit power relationship. This book presents evidence that harboring secrets and the mind's ingenious strategies to defend against awareness may also have injurious effects on the body and physical health. Included are emerging data from psychology on the ubiquity of secret keeping in the population at large, as well as insights from the fields of medicine, neuroscience, immunology, and bereavement studies on coping skills for managing this information to gainsay illness.

The mind has an entire repertoire of strategies for segregating sectors of information. The "vertical split" is one way to compartmentalize a range of feelings, aspects of personal and family history, and sometimes reality itself. We will see how vertical splits occur on a continuum from the healthy to the decidedly dysfunctional and play themselves out repeatedly in secret keeping. The take-home message is complicated. Everyone has secrets, and the task isn't to get rid of them by indiscriminately blurting out everything we know about ourselves or someone else. Finding the tools and appropriate avenues to address this personal knowledge is key, but it is also nuanced and highly individualized.

Over the course of a lifetime, few can avoid hearing disturbing secrets. At the same time, certain career decisions make one prone to hearing more. Attorneys, law enforcement officials, corporate executives, government officers, journalists, members of clergy, espionage agents, and psychotherapists are among the professions who hold the confidences of others. Entrusted with countless riveting stories and traumatic histories, we tend to assume that our training and years of experience inoculate us, keeping our lips sealed and bypassing the signals that might expose us to untoward and unanticipated effects on body and mind. But is this always the case?

Throughout my career and particularly during research for this book, I spoke with numerous individuals who are not in the mental health field but whose professional role includes expertise in keeping secrets. I wanted to comb their brains to find out whether they experienced any impact whatsoever from hearing and taking in so much that must, by the nature of what they do for a living, remain strictly confidential. I was also covertly scouting for tips about how they kept their body healthy and mind sound and avoided becoming overly taxed by what they absorbed from the tasks entailed in the work they find gratifying.

In each chapter of this book, I take up ways to fortify ourselves against burnout and to buttress our awareness of the unconscious aftereffects and somatic reactions that occur when we listen to others. I include some practical and insightful suggestions for managing secret keeping that I learned from my interviewees. Astonishingly, their insights complement emerging data from neuroscience, mind-body medicine, and psychoanalysis.

My own career as a listener to the confidences of others has been a long one. In fact, one secret that I discovered about myself in working on this book is that my interest and experience go much further back in my life than my formal psychiatric and psychoanalytic training! Given the convolution and layering of secret keeping that I contend is so crucial to the psychological understanding of oneself, I believe that it is only fair to share some of this journey with my readers. I begin each chapter with a short personal story or clinical example about how I learned something important about secrets and the vicissitudes of secret keeping. I then delve into the central topic at hand, drawing upon other clinical examples and insights from literature, science, medicine, history, the arts—and, of course, from psychiatry and psychoanalysis.

It only seems fair that a few select patients and students (representing *all* I have had the privilege to work with in many different clinical contexts over nearly five decades) should have the last word. While I thoroughly disguise the clinical and supervisory examples throughout the book to maintain strict confidentiality, psychotherapists learn a great deal about ourselves from the individuals who entrust us with their stories. Patients do, however, tend to keep these perceptions to themselves. In essence, they are keeping some secrets from us *because they are about us.* The withholding usually does not serve them well, but it takes courage—and sometimes encouragement—for them to speak their truth about these perceptions and for us to take in the feedback. Exploring this dollop of secret keeping goes beyond what is usually relegated in professional circles to transference and countertransference dynamics. It's with a sense of fun and pleasure that I now look back and share some of what I have learned from my patients' and students' keen perceptions and sly critiques of my foibles and fumbles that, at the time, were experienced as piercing but ultimately proved enlightening and useful.

This aspect of secret keeping touches on another area that has received little to no attention in the professional literature: why some individuals keep their talents or ability a secret. Their unique skill or innate gift appears to be hiding in plain view. How is the obvious missed, and who fails to see it? Are there ways that therapists can be mindful and then nurture what I suggest are "hidden abilities" that remain concealed until recognized and encouraged by those in the caregiving role? In Chapter 7, I theorize some of the reasons this occurs by employing the fairy tale "Snow White" and an ancient myth, using them as follow-up to pivotal clinical and supervisory examples that taught me much about others' potential that may go undiscovered and, hence, remain secret.

After all the information about the power and burdens of secret keeping, it becomes obvious that personal well-being for anyone in the helping professions requires a place where one can speak openly and ongoingly. Being the confidant of others is one of the great rewards of being a therapist, but we therapists also need good listeners in our lives to stay vibrant and healthy. This nurturing relationship takes many forms. In essence, it facilitates open dialogue about what is often deemed private or confidential. This requires safety, however, and must be earned over time. Those with whom we can share our thoughts and feelings openly ultimately help strengthen our resilience and foster our personal growth.

It is no secret that writing this book has been an enlivening and growth-promoting experience. I have tried to use a conversational style, as if the reader and I were sitting down and in dialogue. Your own associations and ideas, wherever the personal and clinical vignettes may take you—any ideas or stories whatsoever that come to your mind—are important to listen to and to own. You may find that some of the secrets described in the stories are strikingly familiar. You've heard or observed something parallel in your clinical practice or personal life. While we tend to believe that the secrets we hold are unique (and implicitly bad or shameful), there is a surprising overlap of content areas. Secrets are shapeshifters, but there are limits to the forms and patterns they take.

When it comes to secret keeping and confidence sharing, therapist and patient encounter an area of overlap in life that does not always happen. We experience our shared, common humanity. While trying not to sacrifice depth in the professional explanations and theoretical concepts, I hope to create space for thoughtful individuals to reconnect with the pain and joys of undisclosed and shrouded stories that make their appearance in clinical work when least expected, temporarily throwing us off guard but sometimes surprisingly enriching our lives. I end the book with a brief epilogue featuring a few moments from a patient's treatment that crystalizes some of these points.

Secrets tell us who we are, but speaking about them can be extraordinarily challenging. The process stirs fear and internal conflict. I've had to face varieties of both in writing this book, so I assume some readers will too.

The topic itself invites potential rebuke and self-criticism because it implies salacious and dramatic gossip. Other questions arise. *Will I be punished for being a teller of truths others don't want to hear? If someone's world is shaken by a revelation, will it also turn my own upside down? Is serious study of secrets warranted or just plain fluff? When someone else's identity is built on a secret, will it do any good whatsoever to rock their foundation?* I have found that grappling with these questions is another portal into understanding the important role that secrets play in life and why addressing them in the right time, place, and context is both edifying and potentially lifesaving. I also illustrate these finer points with examples from practice, memoir, and literature.

We all hear secrets. We all have secrets. Each one of us needs skills to help us synthesize and manage what we glean from others that is said in confidence. Secrets in psychotherapy are at the heart of clinical practice and a hidden force that shapes human existence in unimaginable ways. We clinicians help our patients and ourselves by learning as much as we can about those secrets and scrutinizing their subterranean impact.

Listening to secrets brings us face to face with the tacit values and tasks inherent in a healing therapeutic relationship. It is an essential avenue to appreciating the strengths and vulnerabilities required to sustain our most intimate and valued connections over the course of a lifetime. In these ways, studying secrets helps inform our clinical work and also guide our lives. Sometimes, secrets take us by surprise because they have stayed sequestered even within the safe confines of a sturdy relationship or within the family context. The therapeutic journey necessitates that clinicians also confront our own secrets. As Freud himself observed, we can only go as far with the patient as we are willing to go with ourselves.

We begin our exploration with a story of a mysterious tidbit of information that popped right out of my mailbox one day at work and led me to undertake this study more seriously. What had I been missing?

1   The Power of Secrets

A folded clipping from *The New York Times Magazine* dropped out of a small beige envelope that arrived in the afternoon office mail. A blurb from "How to Read Palms" explained that soothsaying engages people with questions about their health, profession, and love life. The interviewee was Mark Selman, a well-known practitioner of palmistry in New York City. He made a good living from his art and now provided practical pointers for anyone with the nerve to take it up.

- Gently grasp the other person's hand and be sure to carefully assess each crease and crevasse.
- Study carefully because details you perceive insignificant, such as a scar or manicure, hold clues.
- Redirect questions, especially about longevity, and always leave a sense of hope.

"People will think you know more than you do," Selman opined. "They admit things that they wouldn't tell their own psychiatrists."

The lack of a return address on my mysterious message might have meant that a current or former patient from my psychiatric practice was trying to pull one over on me. Perhaps the clipping was meant to dissipate annoyance or to make a wise crack, letting me know that even palm readers hold more keys to the woes of the human heart than a mere mental health professional like me. By that time, I had practiced psychiatry and psychoanalysis for over thirty years and had conversed with hundreds of individuals. One could say I was just starting the process of life review, undertaking a retrospective appraisal of many privileged moments and personal encounters.

Possibly, a colleague recalled how I blurted out in a moment of weakness that I developed the hobby of fortune telling in high school to overcome shyness (a ploy that eventually worked well as a way to meet people and get dates by college). Surely this couldn't be the roguish wit of my attorney

DOI: 10.4324/9781003471578-2

friend who wanted me to dress up as a gypsy fortune teller to entertain at his forthcoming wedding. Most days, I would have simply chuckled to myself at all the possibilities, tossed the scrap in the office recycling bin, and forgotten about it.

A recent happening caused my mind to lurch down another path; free association is a winding process, after all. Not long before this, I had participated in a forum on career choice at the medical school where I worked. My eyes skimmed over the clipping and turned inward. I was immediately transported back to that meeting in a stained-glass-illuminated classroom. A student asked what had eventually led me to pick psychiatry and psychoanalysis in a field as diverse as medicine. While I wished to be transparent and answer truthfully, I also knew that any major life decision is multifaceted and nebulous; I couldn't do justice to the question with a quip. At the moment, I managed to conjure a plausible answer about finding the practice of psychotherapy a great option for anyone who loves to listen to life stories and finds that doing so has significant healing potential in its own right. Yet my response unsettled me. For reasons I hadn't understood at the time, the unease persisted.

Still fondling the article between my thumb and index finger, I began to recollect my undergraduate career as a dormitory palmist. Engagement that began in the formal parlor with others in attendance expanded to personal appointments in a friend's cozy room. News of my avocation spread. Acquaintances in other dorms quietly reached out to know "exactly what you really saw" about their future and confided that they were bewildered by life.

Gender differences emerged early in the college fortune-telling trade. The predictions riveted women, whereas men dismissed it all as folly and glibly teased that their requested "house calls made behind these closed doors" might circulate around campus and impugn my reputation. Still, I found it not uncommon for tears to flow. I learned quickly to keep Kleenex at the ready.

After the secrets poured, some made me swear an oath never to tell anyone—*ever*—that they were twenty-one years old, a senior, and still a virgin but dying not to be. One brave individual disclosed that he held opposite political beliefs from his distinguished Southern family, had no intention of joining the family firm after graduation, and was dating a woman of a different race that he planned to marry. He shivered as he confided that he was certain he would be disowned for any of these assertions of selfhood because his parents had warned him on multiple occasions about the terms of his inheritance. Why is it that people seek a diviner's counsel and then proceed to spill so much?

Surely it wasn't one of my "university sibs" who recalled it all and reached out across decades to send me *The New York Times* article, a delicate reminder of my promise to keep their confidence forever? Who from those early palmistry days could still be so preoccupied—and so cunning?

Vividly, an episode I've come to think of as "The Suzie Swanky Story" came to mind. After a late evening in the chemistry lab, I had arrived back at the dorm to be greeted by a flurry of my fellow freshmen who rushed to tell me that Ms. Swanky, a beautiful, brilliant campus doyenne, called and wanted to speak to me. "It must be for a palm reading!" they postulated, trying to convince me that just this once I could trust them with whatever it was that Suzie Swanky wanted to know about her future. Although I had not yet perfected the psychotherapist's crafty downward gaze signaling sacrosanct confidentiality, I was sensible enough by this point to deter their voyeurism after Suzie's private session.

Outcomes, however, still beguiled. The resplendent Suzie was not the full package of womanhood that her external portfolio suggested. It took over an hour to still her questions and anxieties about failed romances and her future sex life.

She repeatedly asked me, "Are you sure I will eventually find a husband and get married?"

Nervously, I reiterated my judgment. "See these lines right below your little finger. Make a fist. They actually match up with the tiny islands on your heart line. They tell me you will get married and have a family."

I tried to change the subject and see what else Suzie might have on her mind. I couldn't believe that a campus celebrity would invite me to her dorm room for a cup of tea just to read her palm and tell her what everyone knew to be true—she was destined to fulfill her childhood aspirations of marriage, motherhood, and anything else she wanted to do.

Round and round we went with versions of her same question, as I settled in and attempted to patiently demonstrate, at least by her palm's anatomy, that her future was assured. It wasn't every day that I had the full attention of a college star, and I wanted to make a good impression.

Finally, an exasperated and abashed Suzie blurted a question—as if I had not been paying any attention whatsoever!

"*Well, how can you be so sure when I haven't even...?*" and then stopped just short of completing the sentence. She didn't have to say another word. Her fingertips trembled as she probed my face for expressions of shock.

Abracadabra! Suzie was letting me in on something covertly that she didn't want shared with her peers; she had fabricated a host of stories about her sexual exploits that had made the rounds all over campus. Intuitively, I sensed the secret that was the source of her discomfort and immediately knew I had to proceed carefully without saying anything directly about her lack of intimate contact.

Nothing in all the paperbacks I had read on palmistry prepared me for the impending vetting. While trying to navigate Suzie's questions, I visualized the charts and diagrams I concocted in high school to study palm reading that had earlier proven to be a useful tool in approaching my academic courses.

I took Suzie's right hand and pointed below her wrist. "Just look at your Venus mound. It's right here. Below your thumb. It's voluptuous. Round and prominent. That means you're quite passionate."

Suzie apparently relied on the scientific method, too. She interrupted and asked me to see whether there was corroborating evidence on her other hand to support my claim.

"Yes," I said equivocally, and had her take another look at the marks between her left pinkie and heart line. "Here's where most authorities on palmistry investigate family. These lines indicate you will have two children. That implies to me . . . ."

And then she had me return several times to what I had previously pointed out on her Venus mound. She finally calmed down, but it took another unforgettable twenty minutes of delicately repeating the same points.

I asked whether she had further questions, underscored that all private palm readings were held in confidence, and doused a final sip of Constant Comment tea as she showed me to her door. Time to float away before she asks me to read the tea leaves, too, I silently chuckled.

Snubbed!

The next afternoon, I spied Suzie across the quad and boldly waved as if we were lost friends. I then repeated the gesture cautiously.

Suzie ignored me. Of course, she did.

It took some years before the realization filtered through: when it comes to personal confessions, there are costs to the listener. Few people may actually die of embarrassment, but many flee its reminder. Clearly, the irony had not escaped my newly resurfaced pen pal either. Palmistry: an essential tributary of one psychiatrist's beginning.

The Power of a Secret

What precisely happened between Suzie Swanky and me that provoked her snub and may factor into unforeseen consequences in personal and professional relationships when private details are shared? No one feels good when a friend, colleague, or patient drops us out of the blue. The blame game that can quickly explode further derails opportunity for repair in the relationship because we unsuspectedly become the target of the other person's projection of insecurity and exposure. We aren't privy to what went awry, because the other person isn't about to tell us.

It took me years to realize it, but Suzie's attitude on the quad was likely prompted by feelings of exposure and embarrassment. The successful image she projected as femme fatale on campus broke down during the palm reading as she importuned for reassurance about her future romantic life. To her mind, I held special knowledge that could or would be used against her. She had to protect herself. What better way than acting as if we had never met? As Suzie held court with the bevy of bemused men and women surrounding her, I was simply another annoying interloper.

I never considered that I held such power! Suzie doubled down by acting as if she didn't know who I was, even after we had spent over an hour together that I experienced as bestowing a gift—the time and attention of a palm reading. Of course, I had ulterior motives that were neither secret nor fully conscious to me at the time. Retrospectively, I desired to casually worm my way into a clique of popular undergraduates by reading their palms! When Suzie exposed her anxieties and ignorance about sex, I naively assumed that my reassurances about her future would catalyze warmth and sharing, not sow seeds of vulnerability and contempt that would turn against me.

Suzie successfully disavowed her emotional experience of the palm-reading session by depositing her sense of mortification into me. Psychodynamic therapists and analysts have a term for this process: projective identification. In my youthful readiness to connect with Suzie by spending time reading her palm, I was an unwitting repository for her unbearable feelings of shame. I grabbed the bus to my next class, just sure that I had blown it. Feelings of failure and insignificance welled up, temporarily derailing self-confidence and glossing over another reality. As I read more palms and listened to my fellow undergraduates' reactions, I came to grasp that "hearing" a secret bestows a sense of power to the listener—a power that one must never take for granted.

The unpredictable emotions stirred after a secret is revealed may be difficult for both parties to absorb. A similar process can occur in long-standing friendships and professional relationships. Sources of a secret can inadvertently bump up against us in life, leading to wild currents of emotions and ideas. The substance we must sort through can run the gamut from the insignificant to the destabilizing. These are facets of psychodynamic practice I learned more about as my career progressed.

When faced with stalemate or disruption in a relationship, it's essential to step back and consider all the factors that may contribute. It's equally important to ask yourself whether a confidence or secret provoked pain or shame that the other person decides to sidestep by closing off contact or open discussion. As the meeting with Suzie Swanky taught me, after an individual leaves an interaction feeling exposed and unsettled, an about-face may be triggered. You may get the cold shoulder even though you did nothing consciously to provoke it. Prompted by a sense of responsibility and a desire to understand what happened, on our better days we seek clues about what we might have inadvertently said or done to catalyze the falling out. When something goes wrong, it's common to tumble down a road of fantasy and hypothetical culpability.

After hearing patients' secrets, psychotherapists report experiences similar to mine with Suzie. We might sense that we make a connection with a patient at our first meeting or during the evaluation period. But they might never return. When a well-intended follow-up call or text goes unanswered, we are left in a quandary about what, if anything, to do next.

It's also not uncommon for even the most experienced therapist or psychoanalyst to have a longer-term patient suddenly quit without warning or explanation. There is not so much as a goodbye, let alone the recommended closure process to review the entire trajectory of the treatment. In contemporary parlance, we've been ghosted!

Power dynamics shift in a relationship when one party is privy to information about another that is usually kept private and concealed. This is especially true when information flows one way, such as in a professional relationship with one's attorney, physician, pastor, or therapist. Recall that in *The New York Times* clip, palm reader Selman (quoted in Wollan, 2017) showed his sensitivity to the projection of omniscience and authority onto him. He observed how his clients come in search of advice and "admit things they wouldn't tell their own psychiatrist."

The side effects of confiding a secret even in the safe setting of therapy or psychoanalysis are underestimated. The disclosure may unexpectedly and permanently disrupt the treatment alliance. Psychotherapist Michael Hoyt (1978, 1980) is convinced that the unanticipated consequences of secret sharing constitute one of the most frequent, underreported reasons that patients quit treatment even after a positive start.

The fundamental rule of classical psychoanalysis has been, "Say everything that comes to your mind." Hoyt's observations on secrets led him to modify his technique of inquiry to a more flexible stance. He encourages patients to explore the reasons for maintaining secrecy and urges therapists to cultivate their interest, curiosity, and patience to slowly remove obstacles to speaking freely. Some individuals, he found, solidify their sense of identity by remaining secretive throughout the course of their lives. If they seek out psychotherapy, it's essential for the clinician to explore the motive and function the secret serves and to scrupulously avoid pursuing hidden facts and historical remnants that could threaten psychological stability.

Ignoring me on the quad was the way that Suzie Swanky chose to regain control that she believed she lost and that I could misuse by disseminating her secret. While her active dismissal left me quivering in my loafers, disclosing Suzie's lack of sexual experience as a personal flaw hadn't crossed my mind. After all, I heard many stories just like hers, and, more importantly, I had my own life and problems to contend with.

"The other person has likely moved on," is a perspective I offer to my patients who feel betwixt or disconcerted after revealing a personal story or reminiscence they anxiously regret later. "They don't give it much thought," I say.

> They are preoccupied with their own issues. We get caught up a lot less about what others divulge than they assume we do. Let's try to pull together some thoughts about why this particular disclosure is stirring you up. Maybe there's a piece of your personal history that's important for us to understand together.

In hindsight, Suzie was simply trying to reclaim control that she unconsciously believed she lost during the hour-long session in her dorm room. Other examples in this book further elucidate the leverage that secret keeping and secret sharing hold in relationships, particularly psychotherapy. The old chestnut, "To have knowledge of another person's secrets is to have power over them, a fact of which blackmailers are well aware" (cited in Hoyt, 1978, p. 238), has distinct relevance for psychotherapists who are tasked with helping patients distinguish those secrets that are innocuous from others that are impeding a full life. Timely and judicious disclosure must be weighed against the risks, even if that disclosure has interpersonal benefit. The confidential relationship of psychotherapy is one place to begin sorting through the intangible costs of secrecy in one's life and to decide how and under what conditions to maintain one's privacy.

"May I Tell You Something Else?"

One of my colleagues grew so weary of hearing personal stories and the confidences of others on airplanes that he gave up mentioning he was a psychologist when seatmates asked his profession. In the enclosed, tight space of the cabin, with ambient noise of loud motors running, it's a given that a person who even feigns interest in another is going to get an earful. If you want to learn more about a person, all you need do is create conditions for safety and then actually listen to what they say.

My colleague found that he was better off when he told fellow flyers that he was a teacher (also truthful, because he educates mental health professionals), pulled out his headphones, and began paging through a novel. No one can blame him for not wanting his work week extended and personal space encroached upon. A stranger might easily assume that an off-duty therapist would find their latest crisis or their life story fascinating—and then simply start to unload on them. Another colleague of mine manages to avoid eye contact artfully by staring over the heads of rows of other passengers as she plops down, nonverbally signally her disinterest in conversing. She advises her students, "Listening is our livelihood. It's hard work and a skill set that takes years to cultivate. Most of the time I'm eager to hear about the lives of others but not in turbulence thirty thousand feet above my earthly work!"

Both observations imply a poignant fact of contemporary life. Individuals are not just full of secrets: they are filled with their life stories and often desperate for a place to share them. When the conditions are set for revelation, wonderful and compelling vignettes pour out. It's another tributary to my career choice, even though I discovered it only inadvertently during my years as a dormitory palm reader.

I cherish hearing people's stories. Apparently prompted by the small group readings at parties, peers in college requested private time to ask personal questions. I obliged with delight, closing the door, taking comfortable seats, and dimming the lights to set the scene for disclosure.[1] Questions started, such as: "May I ask you to look at my love lines? Will I get into graduate school?" but soon expanded. It was hard to end a conversation because the content so quickly transmogrified. "May I tell you one more thing?" became a benedictory query, often reiterated until the other person finally let me go. I departed charmed and often moved by the confidences entrusted. I fell in love with listening then, and the love affair continues.

Descending the Spiral Staircase

In psychotherapy, a secret shared is rarely an end to the conversation. This ongoing nature distinguishes the professional relationship of treatment from personal confidences or whispering juicy gossip among friends—or even from partaking in the playful exercise of a tarot or palm-reading session. Those are usually one-off jobs.

The value of a surface conversation of this ilk—one that gives voice to the otherwise hushed—cannot be minimized. It fosters the overarching social fabric of our lives. When one's guard is dropped, it's fine to say a little more to the person on the receiving end. Nonverbal cues such as a tilt of the head, a touch on the shoulder, or a concerned wince signal interest. Trust has been established, and the boundaries of scope and context in the discussion are inferred.

Admit the success you crave; pour out anguish after a breakup; bash an annoying boss, sibling, or demanding parent. You might go as far as spelling out the fantasy of how to settle the score with justifiable revenge if you could. No one is worse off for it. Your secret desires and grievances are now safely deposited with the other person, and you return to your day a little brighter. You may even notice a diminution of body tension and feel strangely relieved, even cheerful. The sense of hopefulness that professional chiromancer Selman believes is essential after catharsis is now restored.

By contrast, the act of telling a confidence in psychotherapy often leads to the revelation of more secrets and personal stories. A gradual deepening of the relationship occurs. Sometimes, an individual is consciously aware that they held information back that they now feel safe to disclose; on other occasions, repressed information bubbles up from the unconscious. In each situation, the end result is the same: new information is available to be reflected on and synthesized over time by both members of the dyad. The sense of self flourishes, and greater resilience is catalyzed.

To describe this iterative process, I employ the metaphor of descending a spiral staircase.[2] My patients observe that they often return to a tale or memory that we looked at previously, sometimes in great detail. They begin to question the relevance of going back and forth, getting into a familiar facet of their life over again. Their plaint is along the lines of, "We have talked this over so many times before today. It's nothing new. You must be bored. I know I am."

My refrain is almost always the same: "But *today* is different. Let's hear the story again and see where it leads." It's not a search for a particular new detail that will unlock a puzzle or expose a secret that springs from this intervention, although surprises may be in store for each of us on the adventure. Every revelation changes perspective and enlarges vistas that will guide the next phase of self-discovery in psychotherapy.

This is the spiral staircase. One retreads similar information—seemingly the exact same story, but each time with different nuances and details. One pauses on the next level of the staircase for a breather. The capacity to be still and make use of contemplative space is absolutely necessary for further reflection and consolidation of gains. Here is where the mastery of old trauma and the integration of painful memories also occur. One reaches a different plateau with each go-round, and it may seem that nothing much is going on. But taking that step and staying on it for sufficient time provides the essential space and pace necessary to appreciate the complexity of lived experience.

The tincture of time does allow secrets that have been withheld— sometimes for decades—to emerge serendipitously or to suggest that the resistances to speaking one's truth have been worn down considerably. After being in treatment for a considerable period of time, it's not uncommon for a patient to acknowledge that "I never told you this before today but . . . ." On other occasions, a confession may be slipped seamlessly into the dialogue and redirect the flow. I'm curious at such intervals to find out whether the details so revealed imply a new level of relational trust or are wily attempts to test my attention!

When the new secrets are broken down, problems that need to be addressed by the patient can emerge. Attention directed to a cover-up is freed, and energies diverted from growth are redistributed. In a best-case scenario, a fuller understanding of the past provides lessons for life from what has gone on before.

Hearing secrets is alluring. The therapist must remain aware of this titillating pull and use good judgment about when and where to back off. Based on his studies of intelligence agencies and public policy makers, FBI historian Richard Gid Powers concluded that less secrecy is usually better than more. A tacit thesis of this book is that adage applies as much to the human psyche as it does to keeping liberal democracy in good working order. Just as "governmental secrecy . . . blighted prudent policy making . . . and changed it lamentably" (1998, p. 20) during the Cold War, so can an authoritarian psyche create debilitating handicaps for an individual whose secrets, both conscious and unconscious, are enmeshed in its webs. Although not intended to go beyond raising awareness of the banality of excessive secrecy in governments, Powers' counsel is ironically fitting for those who tread and pause with our patient on the spiral staircase during psychotherapy. He cautions:

If secrets aren't interesting, nothing is.

(p. 21)

When the secrets were unveiled, what surprises they revealed! But surprises should be unwrapped at the right time and the right place.

Secrecy is a losing proposition.

(p. 58)

An Essential Etymological Essence in the Word

The English word *secret* derives from Latin origins, *secretum* or *secernere*, meaning "to secrete," "(to make) a secretion," or "to separate." Over millennia, the word has taken on many senses, ranging from wishes to conceal, to communicate, to discern, to evacuate, or to set apart. The word *secretion* evokes the realm of the body, with all its liquids, odors, oils, and physical sensations that emanate from within, particularly during sexual arousal. Keeping "all that which must not be mentioned"—human carnality—a private matter is both inferred and advised in the word's derivation. *Secret* is also linked to the Latin *arcanum,* meaning, more specifically, "in need of protection" (Bok, 1983).

Thus intertwined, secrets, the body, sexuality, and their need for protective shielding exert a magnetic force on the unconscious (Gross, 1951). "People are fascinated by secrets," Richard Gid Powers writes. "They always have been . . . Secrecy sells" (1998, pp. 17–21).

In different languages and cultures over millennia, secrecy has taken on qualities that range from the sacred to the intimate to the personal. In all scenarios, a cast is given to what should be set apart and remain within the home. This need does not inherently connote deception or dishonesty. Ethicist Sissela Bok (1983) clarified that all human beings have "indispensable" requirements for privacy. She stresses that privacy is not identical to secrecy.

The need for individuals to discern appropriate context and boundaries in relationships is vital. Beyond Bok's venerated stance, this realization is now supported by developmental research and the psychoanalytic literature described throughout the book. Cultivating intuition and good judgment—all those capacities my lawyer friend dubs "trusting your tummy"—comes down to knowing to whom and how much to reveal in any situation. It's an essential point to remember in our personal relationships and throughout the course of psychotherapy.

As far back as 1919, Freud pointed out that the German word *heimlich* has a dual meaning: that which is familiar, known, and homey, and that which must be kept from sight or the knowledge of others—in other words, that which should remain secret. He was intrigued by his patients' feelings of the *unheimlich*, meaning that which aroused fear and dread, later confessed in therapy. Those aspects of life that are *unheimlich* should also be shrouded and remain secret (Freud, 1919). Because Germans used the words *heimlich* and *umheimlich* in everyday speech, Freud was tying the unconscious affect of anxiety about what should remain hidden to the larger issues of human ambivalence and the repression of opposites.

Language and word derivations zero in on a deep-seated ambivalence. We love our secrets. We hate our secrets. The divergent tensions and conflicts created by secrets cannot be easily catapulted out of our body or mind, much as we want to do so sometimes. Hold them we must. Learning to paddle through the seemingly incompatible affects and the physical burden roused by secret keeping takes a lifetime and is never fully perfected. These twists and turns also create unforeseen riptides for those in the secret-keeping professions, who must anticipate and resist possible undertow from their accumulated force.

What insulation, or protective mechanisms, are available to assist human beings in weathering the universal and inescapable strain that both guards our secrets and helps us know when it's safe—and essential—to disclose one? The answers are multifaceted but hinted at in the case examples in the following chapters. Developmental, psychological, biological, and culture factors all come into play.

One ameliorative ingredient is found in a touching tale of a latency-age girl and her beloved father who sort their way through consternation when their otherwise secure bond is tested. A temporary derailment between them unleashes an opportune moment for age-appropriate dialogue and a necessary pause on the spiral staircase toward adolescence.

A Discovered Souvenir

Eleven-year-old Amy was on the verge of puberty when she and her best friend Joan rummaged through her father's old desk in the basement in search of art supplies. Amy adored her father and treasured the special outings she took with him from time to time. Her idealization came to an abrupt halt when, among all his papers, markers, pens, and paperclips, the girls discovered one unsharpened pencil that read, "Property of Tilly's Whorehouse."

For three weeks, Amy refused to speak to her father. She pouted around the house. Both her parents assumed she was "going through an early teenage phase" of adolescent drama that would suddenly swing in another direction, and she would be her old self again—imaginative, precocious, kind. Nothing mollified Amy's mood or lifted her spirits. Joan came by most days to play but quickly grabbed her best friend and they sauntered off together, studiously avoiding grown-ups and looking unusually serious. Neither parent had a clue what was going on. Finally, Amy's perplexed father decided to have a private talk with his daughter after dinner.

The eleven-year-old maintained her stony silence with the fortitude of a clandestine operative, but her father gently pressed for disclosure. Eventually, Amy teared up and pulled the evidence of infidelity from her own desk. "How could you do this? Does Mom even know you went to a whorehouse? Who is Tilly?"

It was hard for her father to hold back a belly laugh. He immediately understood what had happened and sensitively explained that the pencil was a gag gift that he and some other men were given at a party—a souvenir he had simply tossed into his desk and forgotten.

Amy's father went on to say that he was going to show the pencil to Amy's mother (who, he said, had laughed when she saw the favor a day or so after the party) and would tell her the entire story again if Amy agreed. He was careful not to poke fun at his daughter and make the young secret sharer the butt of a joke. Amy shrugged her shoulders, conveying acquiescence that she didn't mind if her mother knew what happened. In fact, she felt slightly relieved. Amy and Joan, who are still close friends, have reflected on the perceptivity of Amy's parents, who appreciated that even a silly secret held by children can be a sensitive situation. The parents' ingenuousness and receptivity laid a healthy foundation for the now-mature adults to be lighthearted when recalling their youthful discovery of Amy's father's "souvenir from Tilly's."

In this story, the forbearance exhibited by Amy's parents also allowed their daughter to wrestle with her secret discovery, even though they had no idea at the time what she was trying so hard to manage psychologically. By granting Amy sufficient privacy, time, and space to struggle on her own, her parents intuitively provided the safe milieux essential for her to hold and process her conflictual feelings of anger, love, disappointment, loyalty, and letdown fomented by her secret discovery and the aftermath of disclosure.

A child's ability to keep a secret begins around the age of four or five (Margolis, 1966, 1974; Peskin & Ardino, 2003). This step signals a monumental psychological advance in the consolidation of a sense of self. Private thoughts gradually becoming distinguishable from those of others as a child realizes what can be safely held within one's own mind. What psychological researchers now call the "capacity to mentalize" requires that one's caretakers are neither overly intrusive nor abandoning as the child separates and individuates through each developmental stage. In order to keep a secret, an individual must be able to mentalize.

Similarly, the capacity to tell a lie, defined as a "false secret," begins in toddlerhood (Halpert, 2000). Both actual and false secrets may disguise some of the child's tender, erotic feelings toward the parents. Another colleague shared that she was thrilled when her three-year-old son lied about stealing a cookie when she ducked out of the kitchen for a moment. To her, this conveyed that as a mother she was succeeding in helping her son launch and establish a sense of himself. This little boy displayed that he knew precisely what he wanted when she left the room, was finding his own voice, could successfully concoct a fib, and risked his mother's sanction by putting his desire for a treat ahead of his tie to her. The autonomous strivings and cognitive advance of this lie can be encapsulated, "I'll get the goodie myself! No need for mommy! She won't know what happened. It's fun to be naughty."

Less-secure parents overreact to the first lie. They may feel threatened that their toddler is not behaving as they wish or does not need them as much as they did. Messages get conveyed about the risk of having one's own thoughts or taking initiative. Tempers flare that are frightening. Because a secure attachment relationship to adults is also paramount for a child's growth, the normal stages of separation and individuation are thwarted. Derailed by the burden that insecure caretakers may unwittingly provoke, an individual may go on to be wary of intimacy, expecting "intrusion . . . invalidation . . . and betrayal" (Meares, 1988, pp. 653–655) that last a lifetime and can result in psychopathology.

If we remember the power secrets hold, often laden with allusions to sensuality and the body, and the fortitude it takes for the mind to hold onto them, we can assume that, from infancy to the incident described, Amy's parents were neither insinuating themselves into her private thoughts or friendships nor were they threatened by her budding sexuality. They sensed when she was ready to speak and then opened the conversation. By asking Amy's permission to tell her mother, an implicit developmental lesson was reinforced: a secret is not the listener's to share. Amy said her piece, no one poked fun at her, and the temporary impasse was taken seriously by the adults who tuned in. What could have been a derailing moment in development was avoided because Amy's sense of interiority was respected and her ambivalent feelings tolerated. Later, fond, humorous remembrances of the discovery and how it was handled in this family reflect an important aspect of normal secret keeping that distinguishes it from what we take up next: the consequences of what has come to be known from the beginnings of dynamic psychiatry as "the pathogenic secret."

The Pathogenic Secret

When keeping a secret has a decidedly negative effect on body or mind, it is called pathogenic. An individual may consciously hold back an important piece of information or express it unconsciously, symbolically, or by physical reactivity or illness. It is *revealing* the pathologic secret that brings about immediate psychological or physical relief for the secret bearer.

The beneficial effects of confessing pathogenic secrets have been recognized since time immemorial; ancient and primitive civilizations, churches, criminal investigation units, and gifted physicians and hypnotists benefited from the confessional act long before dynamic psychiatrists got into the picture (Ellenberger, 1966, 1970). Despite the diverse circumstances under which a secret may be revealed or exorcised, psychiatrist and medical historian Ellenberger found that the same psychological issues were always at play (Ellenberger, 1966, 1970). What gives a pathogenic secret its power is "the meaning the patient attaches to it according to his personal scale of values . . . he may believe it to be insoluble simply because he does not realize that a solution could be found" (1966, p. 29).

Because they tend to center on a single transgression near the psychological surface, the circumlocutions and disguises found in more complex secret keeping rarely come to light. The clinical examples in this book are usually of this later, knotty variety. Nonetheless, a pathogenic secret is important to recognize because its treatment is simple. The antidote requires of the clinician an ample mixture of sitting still, listening thoughtfully, attending to body language, and, most importantly, calling into question facets of a person's story that don't add up.

In longer-term psychotherapy, the revelation of a pathogenic secret is often the beginning of a drawn-out tale as more history unfolds. Typically, more than one pathogenic secret lies uncovered on the spiral staircase! When one is serendipitously discovered, the nostrum for healing begins with creating the conditions for speaking truthfully and openly about the assumed transgression within the privacy of the therapist's office.

Once the pathogenic secret is said aloud, clinicians are often astonished that the patient soars ahead, particularly when they can divest themselves of stultifying emotions such as guilt, remorse, or shame. Relief may begin on the analyst's proverbial couch, but speaking truth to one's family or community is often a decisive factor for change (Zerbe, 2008, 2016; Zerbe & Bradley, 2018). At that moment, the individual takes an additional and unanticipated turn toward self-responsibility and can get on with their life. "Healing," Ellenberger further explains, "may not depend solely upon the intervention of the therapist, but on the free responsible choice allowed to the patient" (1966, p. 33).

Martin Caldwell, age forty seven, was such a patient of mine. In our first meeting, he told me that his well-established export business went belly-up. He had spent all his savings and was now living off a family trust that was running low. He wanted to change careers but didn't have a clue about what to try. Stalemated, he hoped therapy could help him make a life transition.

In substantial debt, with creditors barking at the door, Martin saw no way out. He admitted that he was disgusted with himself and had severed contact with old friends and colleagues. To top it off, his wife and parents were absolutely perplexed by his shutdown. They grappled with what precisely happened to his business, which had appeared to be doing well. Nothing he told them mollified their questions. His feelings of defeat worsened.

I was fearful for Martin. He was simultaneously dejected and anxious. His life lacked daily structure, an essential exoskeleton for anyone going through a time of upheaval. Despite my attempts to nail down specific symptoms, his eyes darted around my office while he incessantly jabbered. Although he was open with me about his business failure, I sensed there was more to his story. After establishing a follow-up plan for evaluation, I made a few clarifying comments to bridge gaps that emerged in our dialogue.

In four diagnostic sessions, we reviewed Martin's entire medical and personal history. He casually mentioned that his business failed because of cash outlay, excessive inventory, and poor investment choices. I didn't want to raise Martin's ire by seeming suspicious, but I noted how he always circled back to profligate spending and stock snafus as the cause of bankruptcy. Precise in speech and cautious in tone as he calmed during our meetings, he did not seem the kind of man who would be deliberately careless with money decisions. He worried about how he would help finance graduate school for his two adult children.

Slowly I gathered my thoughts and decided to tackle the incongruency. I told Martin that I thought we were encountering two big issues that needed to be addressed immediately before we could move ahead. One was certainly the antecedents of the bankruptcy. Did he understand how he got there? It certainly was not clear to me. Was he holding back specifics from me and his family? There had to be more to the picture. Knowing that the unspoken might not be manifest, I wondered to myself whether loved ones were unwittingly colluding with Martin or had concerns about being direct because he appeared fragile. I said that I thought he was leaving out important details that were essential to know if I was to be of help. In essence, I was circling the back door, preparing for a confrontation that I thought my patient was avoiding by keeping a big secret.

Martin blurted, "How did you guess? Do you feel my anger seeping out from this chair only three feet away from yours? The reason I went broke is not about stocks or stockpiling merchandise. I got embezzled by a woman who worked for me. I thought she was a terrific manager. Turns out she had a huge gambling problem and laundered money through my company. I was a fool to not catch her deceit earlier. What an operator she was! It was an IRS audit that detected the problem. Excruciating! Now I have those steep penalties to pay, too."

I was struck by how quickly he divulged the particulars and wanted to put some balm on his gaping psychic wound. I told Martin, "We keep secrets because we fear that they will hurt ones we love. Let's slow things down and consider all the facts and the pressure you feel right now."

He replied,

> I'm so worried about what the family will do if they know how little money we have. I've eaten through the trust fund. How can I tell anyone that what happened is eating me up too? I'd like to get it off my chest like I did with you, but I know they'll reject me.

I replied that his secret, now disclosed, might be easier to process with friends and family than he assumed and scheduled another appointment.

My tack was to learn more about the situation, to give him time to decompress and muster his courage to be more open in order for me to clarify the feelings of betrayal and rage he held toward the embezzler. I recalled his recriminatory blow that I had intuited his "anger seeping out from this chair only three feet away" and sensed that the heat would soon be directed at me in the therapeutic relationship. I prepared to welcome rage and loathing into the room as the treatment began in earnest.

When Martin returned for his next appointment, he was composed and straightforward. He told me he went home and convened a family meeting. He said he sat down with his parents, wife, and adult children, leveling with them about the embezzlement. He told them he was disappointed with himself for keeping the circumstances a secret. The employee's conduct opened possible portholes into personal liabilities that went beyond the business arena. Was it possible that he was driven by greed that covered deeper feelings of worthlessness? She caught him off guard, he said, and he felt mortified by the layers of malfeasance uncovered during the IRS audit. He knew he had been lackadaisical with oversight. He hated himself for failing those he loved, and any rebuke from them, he assumed, was warranted.

To Martin's surprise, the fallout he imagined didn't materialize. Family members did not shame him. They let Martin know they were concerned and ready to help him reestablish himself in business or pursue another career choice if that was what he wanted. His adult children took more pressure off by telling their father that they would apply for financial help for graduate studies; they did not feel it was Martin's duty to support them. Noticeably brightening in the session as he elaborated their supportive reactions to his truth telling, he concluded, "That's love, doc."

As a therapist, it is heartening to hear all that can transpire in less than a week for a patient who has emotional support. After the four diagnostic sessions, I prepared to take the next step in solidifying our therapeutic contract for psychodynamic therapy. Martin interrupted me in the middle of my offer. He said,

> I did what I needed to do here. I don't want any more therapy at this point. I'll be in touch if I do. What was bogging me down and driving me nuts is clearing. I still feel guilty about what happened but think I can get back on track.

We shook hands and said goodbye.

I never heard from Martin Caldwell again. Our short interaction proved a counterpoint to the Suzie Swanky lesson that opened the chapter. Occasionally, all that is needed for the healing process to begin is for a pathological secret to be let out of the bag. In Martin's case, it appears that the interviews were the necessary gateway to revealing a secret that was damaging him and perplexing his family.

Helping an individual voice their pathological secret and seeing its beneficial effects is a reminder that not all psychodynamic psychotherapy need be long term. A few years after our three visits, I was television surfing. I saw Martin, again a successful entrepreneur and now a self-taught horologist, selling handsome timepieces for men and women on a home shopping channel.

Had he been my supervisor or consultant on this case, psychoanalyst Siegfried Bernfeld (1941) would have found Martin's reactions to be entirely expectable and predictable. In his classic paper, "The Facts of Observation in Psychoanalysis," he points out that a secret is often an important "obstacle to communication" (p. 343) between individuals that, once removed by the act of confession, addresses the core problem. The intersubjectivity created in a psychodynamic consultation is different from that of a structured psychological interview. Spontaneity of interaction moves back and forth between participants, diverting forces that typically get in the way of freedom of thought. Two minds working together in tandem establish the required condition for rapport to build under which ordinary resistances to keeping secrets may vanish. As Bernfeld bluntly put it, eliminating an obstacle to communication by listening "and it alone . . . does the trick" (p. 345).

The Challenge of Secret Keeping

Is keeping a secret possible? Freud didn't think so. After carefully observing his patients and writing about their revelations in his early case studies, Freud explained that the body speaks truths that are often missed during narrative recounting. Based on his clinical interviews with patients, Freud gave us this maxim, which foils the hubris of those who believe their unspoken secrets are shielded by sheer willpower:

> He that has eyes to see and ears to hear may convince himself that no mortal can keep a secret. If his lips are silent, he chatters with his fingertips; betrayal oozes out of him at every pore.
>
> (Freud, 1905a, pp. 77–78)

Espionage agents are among the professionals bound to disagree with Freud, rigorously trained as they are to exquisitely control their bodies and escape foes who are expert in lie detection and sadistic interrogation. Whether the infliction of excruciating pain or isolation from all human contact, torture is known to cause loss of reality testing and posttraumatic stress disorder. Professional spies are likely endowed with unusual brain-based capabilities that foster extraordinary memory retention, cognitive flexibility, and emotional regulation. They may also be endowed with a high tolerance for pain and the capacity to dissociate that effectively shuts down the display of the telltale nonverbal and verbal signals Freud observed in his patients who defended against their hatred, romantic sentiments, and erotic desires by repressing feelings (Freud, 1895, 1905a).

Compartmentalizing intolerable affects or admonitions by loved ones to "never tell anyone, ever" figures into many of this book's forthcoming clinical and literary examples. The strategy requires different sectors and capacities of the mind's defensive operations working in sync to build and maintain the necessary psychic walls to hold back information and sequester it. This defensive stronghold—the vertical split—is costly for the psyche to manage. While it may be effective in certain circumstances (think espionage), it is deleterious in others (think addictions). Essentially, a vertical split relies on the defenses of denial, disavowal, and dissociation to enable a person to keep secrets buried or parts of themselves secreted away from other parts (Goldberg, 1999). In the most egregious and harmful circumstances, the individual with a vertical split is forced to live two lives simultaneously.

With their highly developed skill set built upon natural endowment and the allure of the transgressive, those in the underworld of spying or malfeasance can literally keep their lips sealed and normal body signals silent. Most of us civilians are not equipped to do that, but secret keepers need not be professional spies to recognize that our psyches sometimes partake of similar mechanisms for living with and guarding information. To the extent that we know we are not open books with everyone we meet, we all engage in a degree of vertical splitting. As in a conference meeting room where movable walls allow reconfiguration for purpose, so our own defensive walls go up or down based on need and situation. Appreciating that those walls are to some extent mobile and flexible permits healthier communication and self-integration.

I interviewed a former special ops agent for this book and asked him how he was able to keep his secrets for years after leaving the service. He said, "It's not a problem. The stuff I did—really bad stuff—is something I just don't think about now. I stow it away in a black box in my head. It's locked up." Of course, I attempted to nose my way in further, but to no avail. He shut me down repeatedly despite what I considered to be some well-honed tactics to get his tongue wagging. This contrasted with the man's straightforward and loquacious demeanor in his profession. In fact, I only learned about his prior career because he let tidbits of his past dribble out of his mouth to some of his associates, who then leaked his military background to me in neighborly conversation.

Undeterred, I probed this man for a couple of tips on keeping dreadful secrets to oneself for years without fibbing or divulging or going a little batty. By this point, he was well aware of my interest in secrets and had given his verbal permission to write about our interviews. He also knew I wanted to offer practical advice to patients and readers on "good secret-keeping habits."

I only got as far as his mantra. He admitted that throughout his childhood and adolescence, his father repeatedly told him, "You will have to do things in this life that are hard. You won't want to do many of them. Do what you must and stand by your convictions. That's all that is expected." "So," he elaborated, "I go to work every day. I'm in my late seventies now. Never plan to fully retire. I live by my dad's words. Do what you must do. Be fair. Know when to move on."

A wistful silence pervaded our next moments. His teal blue eyes veered upward, rotating left toward the rim of his straw fedora. He serenely continued, "Such wise tutelage from a man who didn't even complete his secondary education."

Here was the porthole I sought. Staying physically and mentally active while relying upon the voice of his admired father helped this former special ops agent engage in a stealth form of self-hypnosis. He refined an exquisite capacity to dissociate from external reality in the past and was a master at it in the present (Peebles, 2008, 2018). The internalization of his father—and, in particular, his father's admonition to keep putting one foot in front of the other to engage life everyday—worked on several psychological levels, I suspected. The mantra assuaged guilt, alleviating the need for confession of details and helped seal the vault of memory on a need-to-know basis only.

Like some of my patients, but with very different reasons, this former agent drew resolve from a recollection: his father's permission "not to tell anyone, ever, something you had to do." That admonition created the conditions for splitting off unsavory past secrets from consciousness. I wondered silently what would happen if he didn't stay busy with work and why he never considered retiring. I knew he worked long hours, and well into the night too. Was he giving me a clue that busyness is ameliorative for some individuals whose secrets lie behind walls they can never afford to let down? Did hustling and bustling keep those walls in good repair? Would he leak by mannerisms, as Freud suggested, or would past experiences gush out verbally if he had to immediately stop what he was doing, such as becoming temporarily disabled, seriously ill, or sedentary?

This former agent was unfazed when I attempted to briefly sum up recent neuroscientific discoveries, demonstrating just how much intersubjective communication occurs between individuals. I told him that based on contemporary and quickly evolving scientific evidence, more information about ourselves gets through to other people than consciousness alone would dictate. I delicately pointed out that he had spilled a few of his beans to his associates and to me: his work in special ops, stations where he resided during his tenure, his cultivation of natural abilities to memorize and visualize configuration of spaces. His previous life was not altogether secret!

In essence, I was telling the man that Freud was ultimately still correct. A spy or special ops agent might do a better job than most mortals in their capacity to shut down and shut off giving away secret information to others, but they are not able to unplug their body's natural communication system altogether. Secrets can be devilishly hard to hide. Physical reactivity is one mode that betrays this key fact.

In the chapters ahead, the reader will have to decide from the different clinical and research data presented whether enough evidence supports this bold claim. As we have seen in each of the examples so far, a quantum of power resides in every secret held or shared. Those galvanizing effects must be successfully harnessed, lest they overstrain or outstep the body.

The outlet of speaking can stem or propagate the power of a secret. While such release may spawn personal growth, equilibrium is incalculably disrupted when fractures and fissures arising from long suppressed or recently unearthed secrets begin to trickle to the psychic surface. Listeners sit at the edge of these subterranean strata, as the longer example from my clinical and supervisory case files in the next chapter makes unnervingly clear.

Conclusion

To individuals who listen for and absorb the secrets of others, power is bestowed. Confiding a secret even in the safe setting of therapy can unexpectedly and permanently disrupt the treatment alliance. The unanticipated consequences of secret sharing are some of the most frequent, underreported reasons that patients quit therapy even after a positive start.

The ability to keep a secret begins in childhood and requires highly developed competencies for adults whose professional role requires guarding information of others. Likely, different sectors and capacities of the mind's operations maintain the necessary psychic defense structure that enables therapists to be entrusted with much confidential information over a professional lifetime.

The pathogenic secret is consciously withheld information. Revealing this toxic secret brings about immediate psychological or physical relief for the secret bearer and is sometimes all that is needed to help the patient. More often, additional unspoken information pours out over time, so that patient and therapist travel together along a spiral staircase that illuminates the individual's history and personal difficulties. These revelations may impact the body and mind of both therapist and patient, a theme explored throughout the remainder of the book.

Notes

1 Conditions can be adjusted to set the stage for ease of disclosure. These tips about the ambiance of the therapeutic setting are derived from Freud's early papers on hypnosis and beginning the treatment (Freud, 1895, 1905b, 1913). So ubiquitous as to be taken for granted by clinicians of many theoretical persuasions, the usual psychotherapeutic frame and setting was severely upended during the Covid-19 pandemic. As therapists learned during the pandemic, when phone and Zoom sessions became standard practice, the office environment may facilitate personal revelation and resonance with nonverbal communication, but excellent therapeutic work can and does occur under different

and arduous auspices. Still, psychoanalyst Lee Grossman (2023) believes that 90 percent of a patient's communication is missed! Apparently, listening—like playing a musical instrument—requires ongoing practice. To broaden and build these skills, a brief refresher can be useful for the most adroit and attentive recipient of secrets, including therapists. Kate Murphy's *You're Not Listening: What You're Missing and Why It Matters* (2019) is such a guide.

2 The metaphor of the spiral staircase is taken from T.S. Eliot's poem "Ash Wednesday" and elaborated autobiographically in Karin Armstrong's *The Spiral Staircase: My Climb Out of Darkness* (2004). A similar helical model that anticipates the many starts and stops in psychotherapy is taken up in Herbert J. Schlesinger's (2005) *Endings and Beginning: On Terminating Psychotherapy and Psychoanalysis*, who also credits his foundational insight to Elliot's *Four Quartets*. The recommendation of pausing and making time for creative space on the staircase is an elaboration of these authors that I find essential for patients who are trying to come to grips with, and eventually hope to conquer, injurious effects of secret keeping. In our lightening-paced world filled with devices and distractions, it's a hard sell.

2 The Burden of Secrecy

Eleven months after his second grandson was born, fifty-eight-year-old executive Landon Whitehead became acutely depressed and suicidal. His family members had understandably expected Landon to be overjoyed by the new addition. When this new grandpa appeared to unravel before their eyes, they became perplexed and angry.

Landon's constant refrain of "I want to die; I have a fatal disease" led me to undertake a full medical evaluation. He had been admitted to the psychiatric hospital in suicidal crisis. As the attending psychiatrist, I wondered whether this patient had suddenly developed a physical illness that manifested initially as major depression with melancholia. The hospital team members and I smelled Landon's foul breath and musty body odor across the examination room. His ashen and unshaved face, reeking sweats, faltering gait, and agitated moans quickened our customarily methodical workup. Per family reports, he had deteriorated in the previous nine weeks.

In contrast to Landon's alleged conviviality, he became suspicious and refused the visits of well-meaning family members. When staff supportively urged him to talk or participate in activities, he withdrew further. Self-recriminations escalated. I ordered full suicide precautions and one-to-one, 24/7 observation. He frightened nursing staff by repeatedly saying, "I'm guilty as charged. I'm pleading with you—take me out, already." His thoughts always circled back: "You aren't helping me. Life is of no consequence now. A disease is rotting my belly."

When the medical evaluation yielded no physical illnesses to explain his rapid decline, Landon was not reassured. I tried to clarify that his stomach was not rotting, that it was a delusion for us to work on with medication and psychotherapy. Defiantly, he shouted, "I hate you. I'd rather be dead and gone than survive as this miserable beast!"

Withheld for decades, a disturbing family secret was hiding in plain sight, but the blistering particulars oozed out slowly.

At first, Landon rarely spoke spontaneously, whether in individual interviews or group therapy meetings. Head down and eyes lowered, he

DOI: 10.4324/9781003471578-3

routinely rubbed his temples and wrung his fists together. He made no effort to engage with other patients or staff. In addition to prescribing anti-depressant and antipsychotic medications and instituting a specific hourly schedule, I advised Dr. Brian MacDevitt, my postdoctoral supervisee, to try to form an alliance. He should gently prompt Landon to answer big questions that were just beneath the psychological surface: "What do you blame yourself for doing? Why are you responsible? No detail is insignificant. Perhaps you have an idea or 'theory' about yourself that caused this 'dread disease'?" (Zerbe, 2008)

Such direct, detailed clinical inquiry was pioneered by American psychologist Harry Stack Sullivan (1954; Mullahy, 1970) and extended by interpersonal psychoanalysts Clara Thompson (1964), Frida Fromm-Reichman (1960), and Edgar Levenson (2005a, b). To this day, the approach is used to help patients become aware of distortions or lapses in their thinking while concordantly reducing paralyzing anxieties, strengthening self-respect, and promoting psychological growth and a sense of worth. I urged Dr. MacDevitt to lean particularly on the clinical wisdom of Thompson, who believed that a constructive expansion of the self and psychological relief from intense emotional pain and anguish occurs only when a troubled person "finds himself in a less threatening environment than he had previously experienced" (1964, p. 40).

I pointed out to my intern that both patient and clinician draw strength from Thompson's observations that suggest a forward arc in the process of psychotherapy. As she put it, "Hitherto underdeveloped potentialities are discovered and encouraged, resulting in a fuller, more fruitful life." Dr. MacDevitt, who was just launching his career in mental health, found reassurance in Thompson's perspective too: "'he is discovering himself,' meaning that the cramping circumstances of his earlier life are being removed and his capabilities are becoming more apparent" (Thompson, 1964, p. 40).

Patients often have a theory about their own illness that goes unspoken until the clinician asks. Taking the patient's point of view seriously validates and catalyzes the self-reflective process of psychotherapy. Experience has taught me that even patients in dire circumstances often offer up essential but hidden understandings about their lives and how their illness took hold. The psychotherapist's ears are the indispensable tool for a process that cannot be rushed.

Talking to my supervisee, I fumbled over the explanation and shared those favorite quotes that had guided me when trying to establish a therapeutic alliance. Nevertheless, Dr. MacDevitt was a quick study and synthesized the lesson: "Oh, I get what you're saying." He straightened his shoulders.

Your overall approach meets the patient where he is in the moment. It conveys worth and hopefulness. Both patient and clinician need a sense of motivation for growth that happens at every step over the entire life cycle. It reminds me of an aphorism a coach repeated when I was a teenager: *Nobody wins unless we all win.*

Nobody wins unless everyone does? I asked the intern to expand on that. Dr. MacDevitt was introducing his *own* theory of potential curative factors in psychiatric treatment. What he had internalized from a former mentor he would no doubt draw upon over his career. Coaxing along and commenting upon strengths and talents in both psychiatric supervision and psychotherapy, I find, counters the tendency toward self-defeat and creative shutdown.

What the coach said was a revelation to the whole basketball team, Dr. Z. It turned out to be true. We hated to lose any game. It made us practice more. Individual skills improved. Confidence grew. Comes in handy now when I feel competition and envy toward the other interns and residents in my didactic classes—which, frankly, is often.

He laughed. "Then I remind myself—it's my job to figure out my own wheelhouse and run with it."

Dr. MacDevitt grasped that Landon's treatment would require a distinct role and skill set. It would demand the expertise of every member of the interdisciplinary psychiatric team. Within this protective circle, Landon's condition was continuously observed and assessed. Nurses and activity therapists showed interest in him and structured his daily life with projects and exercise. The medications I prescribed decreased agitation and improved mood. Gradually, Landon began to speak spontaneously and more clearly. Dr. MacDevitt and I gathered sobering details during individual interviews and group therapy sessions that the clinical social worker corroborated with Landon's wife, children, and older brother.

All staff members involved in Landon's care met weekly as a team to discuss his treatment plan. We pulled together clinical threads and found ways to remedy our patient's initial symptoms of suicidality, psychosis, and depression. We needed all hands on deck to try to make sense of why this man—who, until recently, seemed to have everything together, and so much to live for—precipitously wanted to end his life and abandon the family he loved, including his new grandson. As Dr. MacDevitt also insightfully reflected, clinicians must continually try to face down our natural competitive and envious comparisons to others to become our fullest and best selves. It's no secret that these struggles are never fully mastered but do lead the way to cooperative engagement with colleagues that shines a beam of light on the patient's needs.

During the first two weeks of treatment, a story emerged. Landon's father had died by suicide when he was a junior in high school. The team social worker reported that the father's suicide had been openly talked about at the time. In a family hospital meeting, Landon's older brother said that their father's cause of death was not kept secret, yet the circumstances that surrounded it had never been revealed. The associate dean at the brother's college compassionately conveyed the crushing news and helped him get home quickly. He was intercepted at the front door by his exhausted, tearful mother who grabbed her oldest son around his chest and pleaded, "Don't ask. I can't talk about what your father did. Not now. Not ever." Team members' curiosity was piqued by this unusual directive.

Other psychological issues would no doubt have been swathed in the hoary emotional cocoon of the surviving parent's command. My professional experience led me to suspect that these would unwind in psychotherapy, but the revelations would take time. The first challenge would be clarification. What had been hidden in plain view, burdening this family for so many years? What particulars of the mystery had stalled the mourning process now implicated in Landon's life-threatening depression? Could the deadlock of unspoken despair be mitigated by psychotherapeutic treatment?

Landon sobbed when he told Dr. MacDevitt what had happened. Setting out to do his chores, he had found his father's bloody body and mangled torso in the barn. He had shot himself in the heart with a pistol. Events that occurred after Landon spotted the corpse were cloudy. Splattered red droplets all over concrete. Pieces of strewn straw. Every imaginable shade of scarlet in the clumps of hay he once loved to smell. Had a rank odor set in already? Understandably terrified and acutely traumatized, the sixteen-year-old ran to find his mother. "My dad was always kind of morose," he confided to Dr. MacDevitt, "but I have no idea why he killed himself."

Landon recalled his mother's instruction to say as little as possible to anyone outside of immediate family. Dumbfounded by the staggering blow, she sought safeguards: "Gossip is going to spread like wildfire in this little town. We must button our lips. Your dad left us with a mortifying mess we will never live down."

Mother then concocted a story—allegedly to help Landon and his older brother, age nineteen, dodge questions. If asked by their neighbors or friends, the boys must follow a script. "Tell anyone who asks," she said, "that your father was told by his doctor days before that he had a fatal disease. Rather than burden us with worry, he chose suicide as a way out. This should shut down the busybodies."

She advised her sons further:

Should anyone have the nerve to try to cross-examine you after that, thank them for their concern. Then say you do not wish to talk further about death. You want to move on with life. You have goals and need to get back to school.

Because Landon, the second child, and his brother were given such clear messages to conceal the truth, they dared not speak forthrightly about their loss to anyone. The unstated message was clear: *Protect Mother. Stay on task. Suppress emotion. Keep sordid details in the family.* Concerns and questions that lay behind the suicide were redirected, another nail in the coffin sealing off Landon's thoughts and feelings. Landon could not mourn his father's death, so emotionally preoccupied was he with keeping the facts of the storyline straight for the sake of his surviving parent.

This situation is different from other kinds of secrets we have discussed so far. Landon experienced the shrapnel of his father's suicide. He had to handle it alone. The discovery of the mangled torso in the barn required another layer of secrecy. For so long, Landon had to find ways to stifle all the residual thoughts, questions, and emotions about what transpired that he was unaware of its catastrophic impact on his well-being. The psychological complications and emotional exhaustion of having to keep a storyline intact become part of secret keeping. The cover-up and details that surrounded the secret, and the ongoing requirement to obfuscate and deny, had taken up silent residence in Landon's psyche all those years.

We Become Whom We Lose

Back at the conference table, Landon's care team began to discuss why the story came rushing in just after his second grandchild was born. Mental health professionals can never be fully certain about why particular events trigger what Freud called "the return of the repressed." Early loss of an essential object tie, such as the death of a parent, reemerges at moments of life transition, particularly when mourning has been blocked (Shabad, 1987, 1993; Warsaw, 1996, 2018). This original laceration to the ego behaves like "an open wound" (Freud, 1915/1917, p. 253) that attaches itself to body memories, metaphors, physical symptoms, and mental pain observed in states of melancholia (Akhtar, 2000, 2001).

The social worker drew the family genogram on a white poster board, vivifying for the team essential family connections and losses. Both Landon and his grandson were second sons. Had the vulnerable teenage Landon been reawakened when he became a grandfather to a baby the same sex and birth order recorded in the genogram? Could the baby's delivery by emergency cesarean section have rekindled traumatic visual and olfactory memories of the original bloody scene? Unwelcome and ambiguous emotions stirred by the birth might harken back to Landon's mother's gaslighting or his sense of his father's betrayal and abandonment by suicide.

I told Dr. MacDevitt in supervision that we clinicians test-drive our ideas in real time by dialoguing with our patient and searching for new clues and ideas that pull facts together. What the patient says *after* we make an inference or interpretation is our collective guide toward deeper understanding. I explained what happens in the normal grief process and that life circumstances—including keeping a secret or maintaining a collusive alliance within a family—can derail this universal, albeit painful, process of working through loss.

Over several supervisory sessions, Dr. MacDevitt and I hammered out what could be happening with Landon. A natural process of identification (e.g., "He looks like you, Grandpa—he's a chip off the old block") usually takes place intergenerationally, but in this case, it sparked a traumatic reenactment. In essence, when the baby was born, Landon's secret that had never been processed was reborn.

His depression took concrete, symptomatic forms as self-blame for the father's demise and wove its way in to a parallel, fabricated tale of having a fatal illness in plain sight. These "identificatory symptoms" (Krupp, 1965, p. 306) are occasionally observed when a loved one dies and there is failure to process anger and yearning. Actual physical symptoms can also appear in the bereaved, suggesting massive denial that loss ever occurred (Gut, 1989; Krupp, 1965; Roth, 2007; Volkan, 1981, 1984, 2007). Landon defended against mourning by taking on the very condition his mother suggested that he should tell others his father had (i.e., a terminal illness).

His identification was so complete that he "became" his father. To avoid additional emotional abandonment and loyally shield family members, Landon simultaneously sacrificed his own need and assuaged his mother's shame and anguish. Through unconscious role reversal and living out the ruse, Landon's psyche attempted to master the original unprocessed trauma—but failed.

While Freud (1921) concluded that identification is "the earliest expression of an emotional tie to another person" (p. 104), contemporary psychoanalysts who study child development have added a complementary perspective, one based on observational research. We know from them that another purpose of identification is the lifelong maintenance of close ties to the most important attachment figures in our lives. These internal representations of others are carried inside each of us and foster a relative degree of independence. In the best of developmental circumstances, we gradually relinquish the other person's presence while taking on, usually unconsciously, some of their attributes, abilities, and interests. We simultaneously feel in our bones that we are autonomous human beings, yet we are emotionally tethered to those we love.

Alongside his clinical concern for Landon, Dr. MacDevitt wrestled with the puzzling complexities that link identification to loss. As he reclined in his chair, I shared that I was reminded of a four-year-old girl whose parents observed that she sometimes took very big steps. She looked gawky and would fall from time to time. My friends had her examined by their pediatrician. The doctor asked the trio to walk around her office as if on a parade. There she noticed what we all had missed—the child strutted just like her father! The pediatrician kindly offered reassurance: "I think this little girl is very fond of her daddy. She's trying to keep up with him. You can see it in her eyes—he's her hero."

Dr. MacDevitt saw the connection. "This is what you mean when you say we become who we lose. Identification evolves from admiration, like this little girl for her dad." I said, "Yes, but also by trying to keep up with her father, the little girl was taking steps away from her mother." Dr. MacDevitt responded excitedly by bringing up the separation – individuation research of Margaret Mahler and colleagues, who emphasized the importance of the rapprochement subphase that begins at sixteen months and leads to the Oedipal phase of development. My supervisee poignantly added, "It reminds me of my own four-year-old son. Dr. Z., he can't wait to play with me when I finish work, but he always shimmies up to my wife after she gets home from being on call."

While identification is another outgrowth of normal mourning, it becomes pathological when attachment for the lost person cannot be redistributed in time to other individuals and interests. Hate toward the person for leaving is redirected toward the self. Sometimes, this takes the form of assuming symptoms of physical disease similar to those of the person who died or weaves its way into their expression of psychiatric illness (Amir, 2008, 2012; Hagman, 1995, 1996; Krupp, 1965; Volkan, 1981, 1984; Zerbe, 1993a/1995, 1993c, 1998, 2008).

Secrets Complicate Grieving

Landon Whitehead's case is consistent with the findings of Krupp (1965), whose patients so strongly identified with a deceased loved one that their symptoms took the exact form of the final illness. Because of Landon's collusive alliance with his mother, painful affects that accompany death such as guilt, helplessness, yearning, a sense of finality, anger, and shame were not tolerated. Concealed from conscious awareness, powerful resistances to owning one's feelings are unconsciously erected. According to Krupp, the typical feelings of rage, longing, and sadness experienced after traumatic loss can be so persistent and excessive that "there is no death, only a change in communication" (Masur, 2001, p. 39).

Some of my own publications have described cases of patients with eating disorders, addiction, anxiety, and depression, who could not process grief following the death of a family member (Zerbe, 1993a/1995, 1993b,

1995, 1998, 2008, 2019). In psychodynamic therapy, my patients and I discuss secreted issues and losses that, once shared, eventually lead to the eventual resolution of the eating disorder. As a teacher, my other professional role, I frequently use examples from practice to illustrate the point and connect them to relevant literature for additional emphasis.

I told Dr. MacDevitt about a female adolescent, admitted to the hospital a few years before his rotation, who refused to talk about the death of her father. Her muteness spoke volumes about unexpressed rage and grief. Team members were frustrated, and their countertransference anger reflected just how much they were containing for the patient. Eventually, I proposed that the patient might have a theory of why she developed bulimia. She pantomimed being the family cat licking her paws as tears ran down her face. She was tending her wounds. Spoken words were set aside for several more weeks as I sat on the floor commenting on the emotions that I saw her embody about the death. I finally was able to connect the dots. I said, "You are speaking with your gestures. This loss is so big, so painful. Everybody in your family is struggling with it, too. It's going to take time." One of Vamik Volkan's (1981, 1984) patients developed anorexia three years after her grandfather died. In treatment, she gained weight through well-established supportive and behavioral methods of nutritional rehabilitation and therapy, but she could never achieve more than the weight her grandfather had been at when he succumbed to cancer.

Somewhat like Landon, each of these cases involves unconscious identification with the deceased that cannot be surmounted until the perpetuated, buried trauma and deep sadness enabled the resumption of healthy development. Essentially, facing these feelings restarts the process of mourning. As I advised Dr. MacDevitt, there is no substitute for the tincture of time in letting go of pathological identifications and gradually consolidating sturdier ones. This is another reason that in-depth psychotherapy takes time: therapists serve as identificatory figures who name and contain painful feeling states long sequestered in body and mind.

When years of secret keeping impede the process of mourning, it's a particularly vexing process for the patient, and sometimes for the therapist, because each revelation brings forth a new layer of personal history leavened with long-suppressed feelings and stored memories that emerge from the shadowlands. The grandson's birth unearthed disavowed family secrets and reactivated the old, unprocessed introject of Landon's father. Had Landon been encouraged to express his feelings of anger, sadness, anxiety, and yearning at the time of his father's death, and to be open about his suspicions and concerns, he would have theoretically been more able to separate from his internalized father and to develop a more authentic sense of self. Other human beings can, to some extent, provide comfort and resources that would not replace the father but could assist in weathering the initial storm and adolescent turmoil.

Landon's feelings had been driven underground: the family history deemed so unacceptable and shameful that it must be sequestered and obfuscated to protect. When that happened, it weakened the patient's sense of reality ("I have a fatal disease"), exacerbated his guilt from collusion ("I want to die... I'm a miserable beast"), and heightened a sense of persecution and self-hatred ("I'm pleading with you—take me out, already"; "Life is of no consequence now—a disease is rotting my belly"). Landon's depression had, quite unconsciously, diverted him from a panoply of unwelcome emotions, family entanglements, and unmetabolized trauma surrounding his father's suicide that were stirred by the birth of his grandson.

Weights on the Mind

Keeping a secret may appear to offer emotional protection for the nuclear family, but it often prevents an individual member, like Landon, from knowing—let alone working through—painful facts and facets of their life. It can also detrimentally impact child and adolescent development. One of psychoanalyst John Bowlby's (1979) most clinically illuminating papers has an apt title: "On Knowing What You Are Not Supposed to Know and Feeling What You Are Not Supposed to Feel." Bowlby found that parents sometimes press their children to "shut off from further conscious processing events that the parents wish they had never observed." "Nowhere," he wrote "does this occur more commonly than in situations of separation and loss" (1979, pp. 405–406).

Based on his years of clinical observations and research on attachment theory, Bowlby concluded that youngsters often shelve memories to comply with a beloved parent's demand. In this case, that was Landon's only surviving parent: his mother. Memory suppression is a strategy to avoid losing love and to assuage emotional pain. Suicidal ideation, severe major depression, chronic anxiety, concentration difficulties, and attention problems are some of the other psychological consequences that Bowlby found among adult survivors who were forbidden to speak their truth about early parent loss and the circumstances that surround it.

It makes sense. When someone tells us a privileged piece of information about themselves, it makes us feel special. It may, in fact, be a gift that bestows particular significance in a friendship or romantic relationship. Who among us has not felt flattered or elevated when someone begins a private conversation by asking, "May I tell you something in utter confidence? It will stay right here, between us, right?" We infer, usually correctly, that this means that our relationship is moving to a new level of trust.

Bonds of intimacy are strengthened after the telling. We listeners may feel a sense of responsibility, but that is a positive trade-off usually managed with few untoward consequences. What is learned in confidence usually elevates self-confidence and a sense of trustworthiness. Most of the time we don't worry about the information slipping out of our mouths either, because it becomes a valued part of the relationship history shared between people who care for each other as equals. The responsibility we feel for keeping the information private is one we take on willingly and lovingly, and hence it is rarely experienced as a burden to bear.

Children and adolescents, on the other hand, hear an adult caregiver's admonition to "never tell" or to "keep this between you and me" as a task they must perform out of a sense of duty that helps them feel simultaneously useful and important. Sensing the parent's vulnerability and neediness, the child secures love and attention by tuning in and complying. It can feel gratifying and ever so grown up to be chosen as a parent's confidant.

Shame, trauma, and competing loyalties after a traumatic loss place the surviving parent in a maelstrom. Safe space is required to have time to think, but in these moments, no place feels protective. We see this in Landon's case. The surviving spouse may believe they have only their child to turn to in the crisis. Grasping at straws just as her world overturned, did his mother assume that she and her sons would be rejected by friends or other families if the truth came out? A suicide can be radioactive in some communities: shunning, gossip, and bullying exacerbate the trauma and the loss of the vulnerable survivors.

No one can ever fully appreciate the pressures and motives that impact another human being. Humility is an attribute cultivated over a lifetime of clinical practice too. It's easy to join the blame-the-parent chorus because an injured psyche will see finding a culprit as an easy fix. In fact, however, life choices and decisions are always imperfect and messy. When we consider what we might ourselves have done when faced with similarly devasting news, clinicians' capacity for empathy and forbearance is routinely tested. In our discussions, Dr. MacDevitt and I reflected on the human dilemma of Landon's mother at the time of her husband's suicide to round out our appreciation of the complex force field that derailed everyone in this family.

Did Landon's mother assume that she needed to protect her husband's reputation? Was she leaning on her children as her confidants and co-conspirators because the suicide gave her a sense of remorse and guilt—feeling states that were simultaneously intolerable and unspeakable? Perhaps even before this tragic event she unwittingly relied overmuch on her children to fulfill the function of partner, friend, or even therapist. If she placed them in a listener role, did that reflect her long-standing empathic failure or narcissistic disturbance?

This burden touches on the issue of parentification of children, sometimes referred to as pathological accommodation (Brandchaft, Doctors, & Sorter, 2010). While our duty as therapists is to understand and support the suffering patient in our care, over the longer haul, we also want to help them to be able to step back and observe—with perspective and empathy—others who did the best they could, particularly under extraordinary circumstances.

When his grandson was born, Landon was given the unintended message that he could neither permit himself to feel nor allow himself to know all that was devastating him. Still unconsciously complying with his mother's emotional needs and demands, he entered the hospital split off from pertinent historical facts that propelled his illness. Mistrust of other people, diminution of curiosity, a tendency toward dissociation, and distrusting one's intuition are some of the additional psychological residual effects that play havoc with individual development when the message is given to the child to close off and shut down emotions, observations, and perceptions of their environment (Bowlby, 1979). This is particularly true when those circumstances involve a primary caregiver.

Fortunately, opportunity presents itself in psychodynamic psychotherapy and psychoanalysis, where patients can safely work through, in a trusted relationship, those details and reminiscences that have been shut away or disavowed. In the therapeutic context, explicit permission is given to speak openly about what one has always "known but been afraid to know." Bowlby cites the example of a twenty-seven-year-old man who sobbed uncontrollably when his analyst followed strands of his patient's associations over two years and wondered aloud whether he had witnessed his mother commit suicide. The analyst reconstructed the history, and a "turning point" in the treatment occurred, "not so much that he was restoring a memory as giving (the patient) permission to talk about something he had always in some way known about" (Rosen, 1955, cited in Bowlby, 1979, p. 405)."

Such wise, practical advice for anyone immersed in the cauldron when attending to another as their suffering begins to bubble to the rim! Cobble together clues, help piece together the storyline, anticipate emerging shards of lacerating emotion, and be steadfastly present to absorb what "weighs on the mind and takes up space in the world" that lifts from the person's shoulders the millstone of long-withheld, crushing anguish.

Sometimes, clinical cases from the professional literature can sound like apocryphal tales, just as they must have to Dr. MacDevitt during that first team meeting, as dubious as a magician pulling a rabbit out of a hat at just the right moment to make the audience gasp in fear or delight. Contemporary substantiation of the impact on the mind of both secret keeping and secret sharing from the field of cognitive psychology offers supplementary evidence and some glimmers into the mechanisms of how and why psychotherapy works. Those who listen to secrets are not, in fact, expected to be Houdini but have ample reason to pay close attention to what is revealed. As chains are unlinked, new puzzles materialize! I now turn to the fascinating findings of two major contributors on the "science of keeping secrets" in the next section to augment psychodynamic understanding of the impact of secret keeping on body and mind.

"An Obsession in a Jar"

Two pioneer cognitive scientists on secret keeping are Daniel Wegner and Michael Slepian. A great deal of psychological research has been done over the past half century on the physical and psychological effects of secret keeping; but Wegner and Slepian's experiments and conclusions have particularly influenced my own consultations and initial therapy sessions with patients like Landon. Their findings also have direct application for anyone whose clinical practice involves keeping secrets, from novice psychotherapists to well-seasoned psychoanalysts. I routinely reference Wegner and Slepian when I teach those entering the mental health field and when consulting with anyone whose profession involves preserving confidentiality.

One of Wegner's most famous experiments is colloquially referred to as "The White Bear." In the original 'White Bear' study, in the late 1980s, Wegner drew upon an old Russian folktale of a man who tells his younger brother to sit down and to *not* think about a white bear (Lane & Wegner, 1995; Wegner, 1989; Wegner & Schneider, 2003). As it turns out, the man discovers that his brother can think *only* about the white bear, the exact thing he is *not* supposed to think about. Wegner wondered whether the fable picked up on something significant about the real-life psychology of human beings. He set out to see whether keeping a secret can have incapacitating effects on the ability of humans to think our own thoughts and stay clearheaded.

Ask someone to keep a secret—like a juicy piece of gossip or morsel of a tantalizing story—and see just how hard it is! Wegner suspected that it would be more difficult than it seems. He was right. When asked *not* to think about a secret or keep a piece of information to oneself, in our minds, it becomes just like the fabled white bear. His experiments demonstrated, time and time again, how impossible it is to turn off even an innocuous thought and not think of anything else.

For example, Wegner selected two groups of college students as subjects and asked each group to say everything that came to their mind into a tape recorder for five minutes (Wegner, Schneider, Carter, & White, 1987; Wegner & Zanakos, 1994). One group was told to think of anything *except* a white bear, and the control group was told to think anything, even the white bear. Whenever an individual in either group thought about the bear, or mentioned it, they were instructed to ring a bell. The subjects who were told to suppress thoughts about the white bear rang the bell considerably more often than those who were told that they could include them. There was even a rebound effect: when released from their task of thought suppression, the subjects who had been instructed to keep the white bear out of mind poured it out verbally more often in the follow-up interviews than the control group did.

When asked to guard a piece of information, individuals sometimes displace the unwanted thought onto an object in a room to get rid of it. This creates a new and annoying problem. A bond forms between the unwanted thought and an object. The difficulty in stopping thinking about unwanted thoughts now multiplies and expands. Wegner concluded, "We don't realize that in keeping it secret we've created an obsession in a jar" (Jaffe, 2006; Wegner, 2011). We might think of Landon and his bottled-up obsession.

Wegner's research builds on studies of human perception known as dichotic listening. Human brains protect us from sensory overload by tuning out of all kinds of information, allowing us to focus on the most important details that we actually need. Psychoanalyst and researcher Emanuel Peterfreund expanded our understanding on this type of selective attention in his experiments on auditory messages sent simultaneously to both ears of his subjects (Peterfreund, 1971, 1972, 1980, 1990). When he asked one subject to listen to and repeat a message given to the left ear only, the individual could easily comply. By contrast, if a personally significant word, such as one's own or a significant other's name, was uttered in the other ear, he was distracted and found it more difficult to comply. Peterfreund's discovery nuanced our understanding of "subliminal perception," which had been studied for decades. Human beings can selectively attend to or shut off messages from conscious awareness while believing that they are dialed in to the full gist of the conversation.

The implication for individuals is clear: we have much less control over the information that we take in and how it influences us than we think. A person who is holding on to a completely benign piece of information might get tied up in knots without even being aware of it. We can't shut it off. Think of planning a surprise trip or buying a special gift for a loved one. You are excited about the plans or the gift. The harder you try *not* to think about it in their presence, the more it seems to slip through your lips.

Michael Slepian, a professor at the Columbia Business School, and his colleagues also concluded that it's hard for people who are told a secret to keep it off their minds. Their research illuminated that most people are keeping an average of thirteen secrets in one of thirty-eight categories, such as infidelity, surprises, abortion, and illegal behavior (Slepian, Chun, & Mason, 2017; Slepian & Greenaway, 2018; Slepian, Kirby, & Kalokerinos, 2020). Joyous secrets, such as early pregnancy or a budding romance, are equally hard to hold. The more deliberately and actively individuals try to conceal secrets, the more it seems the mind wanders back to them.

Slepian and colleagues found that shame, rather than guilt, is the primary negative emotion associated with secret keeping. The amount of time spent thinking about the secret takes an additional toll, particularly when it is associated with negative emotions. Slepian concludes, "When you feel guilty, you can make amends or decide to do something different the next time... Shame (makes) you feel helpless and powerless" (Weir, 2020). Feelings of helplessness are a prime factor in leading a person to rehash secrets over and over.

All the more reason to wonder about the buildup when secrecy occurs over a longer period of time, and not under the controlled experimental conditions (i.e., in the "real" world) of a psychological investigator. With hard data provided by studies such as those of Wegner and Slepian, therapists have an additional armamentarium to ground our patients, anyone in a secret-keeping profession who consults us, and ourselves.

It's a matter that Dr. MacDevitt and I discussed as well. We clinicians are privy to all kinds of private information over the course of our career and are just as likely as anyone else to glide over the accumulated debris. It builds up. Is there a tipping point that contributes to burnout for anyone with secrets to hold, including psychotherapists?

Weights on the Body

Here and throughout the book, I suggest that any deleterious impact of secret keeping can be attenuated by raising conscious awareness and by applying some individualized self-care tools in the here and now. (This becomes very important in Chapter 5, on somatic countertransference.) I think of these unintended negative consequences of secret keeping on body and mind as "the burden of secrecy." While it's an essential task of the therapeutic relationship to hold and contain the confidences of our patient, it's also an obvious area of overlap of life experience that both patient and therapist share; each must learn to constructively manage the "side effects" of keeping secrets.

Most of the time, the secrets we keep to ourselves, about ourselves, and for others don't create an "obsession in a jar." In fact, they might never come to mind at all unless something or someone brings one to mind, and thus they rarely "take up space" in our world. This minimal impact shifts momentarily if a chance encounter or repressed memory brings the stowed away to consciousness. Then we have the task to imagine what to do next, if anything at all. It's a common occurrence in daily life that weaves its way into conversation in relationships, teaching, and psychotherapy sessions.

Individuals often ask how a psychoanalyst goes about holding so much private information about others for years without letting the cat out of the bag.[1] As you can imagine, this has become a particular topic of inquiry in my practice since I began writing and speaking about the topic. I notice that advice is surreptitiously sought about how to recognize and cope with the "secrets of everyday life" that one knows must be kept under wraps to avoid harm, exposure, and embarrassment. As a prompt to remember the dilemma we all face in keeping confidences over the course of a lifetime, I suggest an unsavory visual analogy: contending with a complicated, conflictual secret is akin to discovering an unexpected tiny wart on one's finger or toe. I call these sneaky emotional eruptions "psychic warts" because they are rarely dangerous but can be annoying and sometimes need a little tending with reflective thought (Zerbe, 2019).

A typical example goes something like this. You are out with your spouse or colleague and run into someone who knew you "back in the day," when you made the rounds at the Burning Man desert festival. Each of you has some private goods on the other that are relatively innocuous, but you prefer they not be shared. You're puzzled by your ambivalence about this chance encounter and bugged by the unanticipated physical aftermath. The extra beads of sweat dampening your brow and armpits, that nervous giggle of complicity, and the full-throttle trot to get away after you say goodbye (which your companion doesn't even notice) all signal your autonomic nervous system at work. You splutter and snicker but keep moving, puzzled by the admixture of pleasure at seeing your old buddy and the desire to get away as quickly as possible.

Given a harmless situation, think of this alert as your body's physiology running a routine maintenance check. Your early warning system told you to get away from an agent of stress! Neither you nor your old friend has had your cover blown by the incident. Your silent reminiscences are totally safe. The fact that your body simmers down after you order a whiskey sour or duck into the movie theater is all you need to remind yourself that the danger of exposure has passed. It all happens within microseconds. You can even reassure yourself after the fact that your neurobiology's early warning system is in good working order. But, in my parlance, you just stumbled onto a psychic wart.

Sticking with the metaphor, it's quite rare for warts to become cancerous, but a few do warrant sustained observation. The psychic and corporeal fallout of concealment can be tricky to gauge because it occurs on a continuum from the truly innocuous to the decidedly malignant. Tolerance for ambiguity and fortitude in the face of human frailty are highly individualized capacities, and children and adolescents have far less ego strength than adults to weather these strains. What might be only a psychic wart for an adult to manage may cause long-term damage to a youngster.

Concomitantly, psychic warts accumulate over the years. These layered emotional encrustations take circuitous paths along the conscious/unconscious continuum and may announce themselves in later psychiatric problems and interpersonal derailments, as we discover in this book's case examples.

When Landon Whitehead was asked by his mother to keep the details of his father's suicide a secret, he was placed in an impossible position. Despite his later accomplishments in business and family life, the onerous role of confidant took enormous emotional energy that kept Landon's entangled ruminations about the details of the suicide alive for years. They weren't always on the tip of his tongue, but they smoldered in the background.

Like the titular adolescent character in Stephen King and Richard Chizmar's bestseller *Gwendy's Button Box*, who hides, cares for, and never mentions to anyone the special box she is given by an interceder, a youthful secret keeper often questions why they were the one picked for the task (King & Chizmar, 2017). The lens of fiction enables readers of the novella to experientially tune in to the protagonist's plight that echoes what we overhear in practice from adolescent and adult patients. King and Chizmar write of the adult protagonist looking back: "Gwendy has a thought: secrets are a problem, maybe the biggest problem of all. They weigh on the mind and take up space in the world" (pp. 29–30).

The physical consequences bedevil Gwendy now as they did in her teens. She "worries" (p. 49), hears "a constant hum" (p. 49) in the head, notices a "little voice inside (who) is asking questions" (p. 65) like "what is it doing to me" (p. 66), and "thinks about it... but wants nothing to do with it" (p. 126). These apt descriptors link body and mind to the psychic injury that imperils an adolescent with a big secret to hold, one that takes up too much "space in the world" and commonly constricts emotional and cognitive development.

Recall how Landon arrived at the hospital emotionally and physically exhausted, unable to process information, pale and downtrodden. Although the treatment team knew only the bare bones of his story at that moment, the telltale signs of illness were visible to everyone. It's conceivable that his physical delusion may have been one additional sign of a benighted constitution and corporeal peril. In Landon's case, years of secret keeping were the proximate cause of severe stress that disrupted his body's homeostasis and contributed to severe depression and suicidal preoccupation.

It's reasonable to wonder how the phenomenon of secret keeping impacts the body and wreaks so much havoc on the mind. I maintain that when the "burden of secrecy" is prolonged and severe, the same neurocircuitry that regulates arousal, neuroendocrine, and affective responses within the hypothalamic-pituitary-adrenal (HPA) axis is at risk to derail. In effect, the original trauma of his father's suicide threw into overdrive Landon's autonomic nervous system, which regulates stress and is one of several "distinct emotional systems" (Panksepp, 2009; Panksepp & Bivens, 2012). The finally tuned balance between the sympathetic and parasympathetic systems was worn to a frazzle over many years by the ensuing propagation of his family's false narrative and counterfactual script.

Twenty-first-century neuroscience is tying many invisible, body-based feedback mechanisms to psychic injury. A breathtaking array of laboratory and radiological tools such as fMRI and PET scans lifts the shroud on what precisely transpires in the brain that leads to the near demise of a patient like Landon. The mechanism I wish to emphasize in this chapter is the HPA axis because it is the most well researched to date and links stress to psychiatric disorders that are themselves comorbid with numerous medical conditions: coronary artery disease, some cancers, diabetes, hypertension, and chronic inflammatory diseases such as colitis, gastritis, and hepatitis.

Excessive stress of the magnitude Landon faced leads to hyperactivity of the HPA axis via secretion of hormones such as cortisol, vasopressin, and corticotropin-releasing hormone. Mounting evidence also suggests that abnormalities in the HPA axis are associated with depression and cognitive impairment due to increased secretion of cortisol and insufficient inhibition of the glucocorticoid receptor regulatory feedback mechanisms. The primary inhibitory neurotransmitter acting in the paraventricular nucleus of the hypothalamus, gamma-aminobutyric acid (GABA), is also affected by stress and is likewise implicated in HPA dysfunction. A comprehensive medical workup at the beginning of psychiatric treatment such as Landon's is undertaken to rule out a medical problem that presents as physical disease *and* to scope out the downstream effect of years of stress-induced neural dysregulation that may be ameliorated in part by psychotropic medication and psychotherapy.

Adding to the findings of Slepian and Wegner, contemporary biology offers a new vantage point on the accumulated repercussions of secret keeping implicated in physical and psychological breakdown. As described by Bowlby, some of the outward manifestations of "knowing what you are not supposed to know and feeling what you are not supposed to feel" are compulsive and recursive thinking, inflexibility, inhibited cognitive capacity, and emotional constriction born of insecure attachment. We now appreciate that gaslighting overtaxes the psyche and impacts the brain's physiology similarly to other forms of chronic trauma: to keep the concealed information sequestered, the same neurocircuitry comes into play. Ultimately, markers of inflammation change. Metabolic dysfunction occurs. Even brain tissue atrophies, diminishing the capacity for cognitive flexibility and resilience over time. Physical disease becomes more likely because the immune surveillance system's response is also taxed. Clinicians must knit together some of these perspectives into the treatment plan to address the high cost of secret keeping. For people like Landon, secrets take up enormous space in their world and eat away at their very selfhood.

Why Now?

In supervision, Dr. MacDevitt struggled to formulate other reasons that may have contributed to Landon's depression at this moment. It's the same question concerned individuals and experienced clinicians frequently ask: "Why did this crisis occur now? It erupted without warning. It still makes no sense. He was high functioning and running full throttle. He appears to have everything he ever wanted."

As I reiterated to my supervisee, clinicians are always puzzled by what brings about sudden decline and life-threatening symptoms at any age. We can never be fully certain of the full etiology. Psychiatric illness is multidetermined by biological, social, and psychological factors. Hints do appear, however, and often we need not look far to make some useful conjectures to launch treatment.

Times of life transition are particularly ripe for a tumultuous backslide, an upsurge of emotional exhaustion, and the neurophysiological dysregulation we see in Landon's history. Developmental passages temporarily turn our internal object relationships and interpersonal connections with other people topsy-turvy and inside out. For everyone, the "internal furniture" of our intrapsychic home must be updated and rearranged to meet the demands of a new epoch. Successful negotiation of earlier developmental transitions is no guarantee that the next will occur smoothly, although emotional muscles (Novick & Novick, 2010) that were shaped and strengthened early on are called on again in subsequent life phases to reengage and master new challenges.

When patients can step back and begin to ponder what befell them and consider in collaboration with the therapist different hypotheses about what happened, they are on the road to recovery. When secrets and secret keeping are part of the picture, we might liken this process to the additional fortitude it takes each of us to look inside the black box of the concealed stories we keep from others that has significance for ourselves and for them. We must also confront existential queries we usually keep to ourselves, or at best utter under our breath in moments of private kvetching: *Why did this happen to me? Is this my fate?* The void of unfathomed personal history or expectant tumult lies secluded in the backwaters of our grievance and kept under wraps in conversation to avert the appearance of self-indulgent commiseration. A therapist's interest pierces that void.

Individuals must answer these anxiety-packed queries: *What have I been keeping from knowing about myself that is important to acknowledge to move forward? Do I have some secrets that serve defensive functions that are no longer useful? Are they setting me back in ways that I hide from myself and loved ones? Am I comfortable with the limits, boundaries, and level of privacy I set in relationships?*

Focus shifts to the patient and his story rather than on the more equitable back-and-forth that happens dialogically in other relationships. It's this speaking-together between therapist and patient about the caustic, upending, and heretofore submerged facts and feelings that elicits the dominant features of the suppressed secrets that will eventually provide the salutary balm of healing.

Dr. MacDevitt and I discussed how Landon's depression at age fifty-six exhibited many features of a severe midlife crisis. Until this point in the life cycle, he had been able to ward off depression by being thoroughly capable and competent at work and in family life. He was, in the words of psychoanalyst Eliot Jacques, "a doer" who could seemingly put to the side his father's suicide, his mother's needfulness, and all those ramifications of the disguised pact made in the family from adolescence through middle adulthood.

Middle age demands taking stock of personal achievements and limitations, coming to peace with them, and contemplating one's own death. This is a difficult transition for most, but impossible for someone with a faulty foundation like Landon's. His adolescent development, inherently a time of transition and turbulence, was scarred by the premature death of his father, the horrific, blurred circumstances surrounding the death, and his mother's ongoing demands for camouflaging. This meant that Landon lost normative parental provisions and had the additional responsibility exacerbated by role reversal—the caretaking and emotional squelching required by his mother.

The layers of concealment discovered early in treatment were the tip of an iceberg. Landon had no role models for health aging. He was emotionally impoverished by the lack of internalization of good objects. By the time he made his way to the hospital, he was ruled by his bad internal objects, which unconsciously and enviously competed with his newborn grandson, whose birth represented not only a generation that would eventually succeed him but, in the present, would receive the parental love and care he still craved.

When hospitalized, Landon had already surpassed his father's age by more than a decade. In many respects, his life had flourished despite the trauma. However, conflict is stirred for anyone who lives beyond the lifespan established by a parent. While starkly facing one's eventual demise, the survivor must now paradoxically own that they did not succumb as their parent had. Guilt must be faced down to preserve generational continuity, but it is painful to simultaneously own having gone further than the parent and missing out on their longed-for love and approbation simultaneously.

Elliott Jaques (1965) clarifies that unless good internal objects are well established and sturdy, "unconscious depressive anxieties are aroused . . . (and) death itself is equated with depressive chaos, confusion, and persecution" (pp. 510–511). Each of these clinical features—depression, chaos, confusion, persecution—is observed in Landon's case history, reflecting a paucity of suitable internal objects to rely upon, soothe, and point the way forward in middle age.

Family secrets complicate the normal process of adolescent separation and individuation under any circumstance (Avery, 1982; Jacobs, 1980; Richman, 2009). At an age when the teen should be taking steps away from the family and negotiating the core conflict between wanting to stay and yearning to be on one's own, secrets keep the child bound. To some extent, skeletons in the closet can be split off from conscious awareness and displaced so that the façade of an ideal family is preserved. Further loss is forestalled by loyal concealment, but at the expense of expressing one's autonomy. Mourning is also postponed (Avery, 1982; Warsaw, 1996, 2018).

As Landon's history demonstrates, the brothers sought to spare their mother and therefore colluded with her in not speaking the truth. In this process of mystification, a youngster learns not to fully trust their own mind (Jacobs, 1980; Richman, 2009). Eventually, however, the organizing function of secret keeping breaks down because the individual can no longer collude with the false family narrative. Guilt, resentment, aggression toward the self and others, repression of libidinal drives, loss of vitality, fragmentation, and episodic dissociation are other symptoms that press on the individual and lead them to treatment, seeking solace and a witness to help them make sense of their narrative.

Based on her experience as a hidden child during the Holocaust, analyst and author Sophia Richman (2009) has found that multiple attempts at therapy may be necessary to expose layers of secrets that leave "an indelible mark" (p. 67). A full reconstruction of their toll may not occur until middle age. Encouraging other analysts to self-disclose as a role model for others, Richman found writing to be a remarkable additional resource in constructing a fuller narrative of her life after two prior experiences in psychoanalysis. Yet with respect to her personal history of sequestered secrets that could not be spoken about in her family even years even after the war, she shares that she found it essential to

> Face the fragmented past with the help of an empathic listener . . . to recognize the impact of my childhood trauma . . . [to explore] their

meaning and their lifelong impact . . . [and to create] a narrative that made sense and felt authentic.

(pp. 68–69)

Landon's Psychotherapy: First Steps in Recovery

After the initial witnessing and validating suggested to help the patient establish a sense of safety and settle into treatment, it was the task of Dr. MacDevitt and me to help Landon observe and challenge his "obsessions in a jar" and educate him about the corrosive effect they likely had had on his mind and body over the years. We did not want to take away this defense so much as to get Landon's attention so he could begin to make constructive change by creating conditions of safety (Allen, 2022).

We based our plan for Landon in part on the writings of psychoanalyst Bernard Brandchaft (1985, 1988, 2002; Brandchaft, Doctors, & Sorter, 2010; Stolorow & Brandchaft, 1987), who called the psychotherapy process "emancipatory" because it challenges long-held patterns of pathological accommodation (2007; Brandchaft, Doctors, & Sorter, 2010). In his practice, Brandchaft treated patients like Landon with severe depression and obsessional disorders who did not make sufficient gains with either medication or previous psychotherapy (Brandchaft, 1988, 2001, 2002; Brandchaft, Doctors, & Sorter, 2010). He found that their obsessional symptoms could be traced to an unconscious symbiotic relationship with a caregiver. Patients relented to their obsessions when they tried to detach themselves from their caregivers' needs and attempted to begin to live their own lives. Implicit is the notion that the patient is not allowed to think their own thoughts because they are emotionally preoccupied with attuning to the needs of the other person, on whom they also depend. A layered family secret and gaslighting are sources of such symbiotic enmeshment.

Based on years of acquired clinical evidence, Brandchaft concluded that something went terribly awry in the attachment patterns for such children and adolescents in the home. The patient was listening to his caregivers, but no one was listening to the developmental needs of the patient. The caregiver had both conscious and unconscious conflicts that they turned to their child to solve. The child cannot meet these demands, resulting in self-hatred, craving for attention and understanding, and compulsions brought about by "the profound feelings of worthlessness and despair in one's utter failure to have brought joy into the lives of caregivers" (Brandchaft, Doctors, & Sorter, 2010, p. 174). Landon's loyal efforts to assist his mother were considerable, but ultimately insufficient. He could bury the information he had, but as an adolescent boy, he could neither solve his mother's problems nor bring her delight.

Building on the research of Bowlby and others, Brandchaft observed that obsessions serve a protective function for the self. Obsessions are a co-created unconscious defense that maintains the attachment between child and caretaker. This child—the patient-to-be—essentially diverts their psychic energy and libidinal drive to care for the parent. Those "obsessions in a jar" that begin with secret keeping have cognitive, biologic, and psychodynamic roots that in extreme form yield the kinds of psychiatric illness that afflict individuals like Landon. Development of the self is neglected. In this context, circular and compulsive thinking arise from the child's relentless striving to attune themselves to the caretaker's needs.

Maintaining contact with their unhappy, depressed caretaker is lifesaving for the child. Guilt and shame inevitably arise because of the failure to meet an adult's needs. Brandchaft and his colleagues treated many patients like Landon who tried to maintain the therapeutic alliance by caring for or attuning to their therapist's well-being, just as they had done for their parent. Patients repeated this pattern multiple times in the transference process, where it could be observed and interpreted. The clinician-writers who worked under the tutelage of Brandchaft discovered that the obsessions served a dual purpose for their patients. The patients could turn away from their own perceptions and desires and simultaneously carve out and maintain the attention of the therapist.

Our task as Landon's treaters was to help him see that the secret keeping was all about his attempt to tune in to the needs of his mother at the cost of suppressing his own thoughts and self-assertion. This "system of pathological accommodation"—a term eventually coined by Brandchaft—is inevitably repeated in the psychotherapeutic relationship, and clinicians must persevere in our attempt to go behind the veneer of compliance. This "preordained purpose to bring happiness to the lives of its unhappy caregivers" (Brandchaft, Doctors, & Sorter, 2010, p. 186) is subtle and recursive. The patient's finely tuned antennae continually search for the wavelength to reach the therapist, trying to anticipate the response she wants. Consequently, change "is for the most part silent, slow, precarious, emergent, and incremental" (p. 165).

Viewing the secret keeping, depression, and obsessional consequences as a profound failure in Landon's adolescent caretaking environment, psychotherapists set out to help understand why an individual would nullify his own perceptions at every turn. Whenever he disagreed or shared an idea of his own, Dr. MacDevitt and I welcomed Landon's point of view, but we were aware that he might simply be trying to appease us. False compliance is expected in the early stage of therapy for people like Landon who have been astute caretakers for their parents or siblings and must be gently confronted. We wanted him to share his truth—that is, to begin to let us know what he knew and what he felt that was real as a series of first steps in building a truer sense of himself.

With a jest that insinuated a larger educative purpose, I told Dr. MacDevitt,

> When it comes to Landon, my favorite words to hear him say are, 'No. You're wrong, Dr. Z.' That's when we clinicians get a little closer to knowing that a patient such as Landon experiences us as separate people who can survive disagreements—even their disagreeableness. It's a sign that they are less afraid to step on our toes. They aren't taking care of us. They don't have to keep their anger and disappointment a secret either.

The intervention has an additional purpose. The normal turbulent period of adolescence, during which the second separation-individuation process occurs (Blos, 1962, 1979), had gone off track for Landon. Psychotherapy cannot turn back the clock and reverse horrific events, but it can promote maturation and the development of ego functions that were blocked by an original trauma. Independence of mind and healthier separation from internal objects were furthered when the team encouraged and valued Landon's differences and did not retaliate when he spoke his mind. The adolescent tasks of superego reorganization and the establishment of ambivalent object relations, so essential for adult living, could then ensue. Landon would no longer submit unconsciously to his mother's dictates and her falsification of reality.

Another Rung on the Spiral of Healing: Provision of Social Support

Concurrent with the individual therapy, and as the layers of secret keeping became more accessible to Landon, team members provided the social support necessary for the mourning process to restart and, to some extent, be worked through (Allen, 2002; Gut, 1989). Their felt presence surrounded Landon. Team members were sensitive to the patient's shifting affect states and normalized the experience of grieving, much as a community of mourners does for any bereaved individual. In fact, Landon decided to create his own ritual by making a small wooden box in activity therapy where he stored "my file of private thoughts about Dad" as they made their way back to consciousness.

When he was ready, he buried these slips of papers in a rose garden, accompanied by his three favorite staff members. It was a surprising but simple gesture in letting go of his internal stockpiles of silenced thoughts and questions, advancing the mourning process within a small community of grievers (witnesses) simultaneously. In a team meeting near the end of hospitalization, we conceptualized how Landon was making use of the "good objects" he could now internally embrace. He was allowing us to mourn alongside him, potentiating our own growth as treaters and human beings who ourselves experience losses over the course of life and must also take time and space to grieve. Together in team meetings, we referenced Melanie Klein's (1940) perspective on the importance of community in moving through a mourning process more than once:

> If the mourner has people whom he loves and who share his grief, and if he can accept their sympathy, the restoration of the harmony in his inner world is promoted, and his fears and distresses are more quickly reduced.
>
> (p. 145)

Moral Injury: An Additional Concept to Assist the Patient

Psychoanalyst and researcher Jane Tillman, an expert in the psychodynamics of suicide, includes the concept of moral injury to assist survivors of parental suicide like Landon (Tillman, 2016). She points out that in addition to the essential reworking of identifications and object relationships that occur after any death, the parent who suicides abandons the child and "his or her moral authority regarding the endurance of love, hope, and the basic value of life" (p. 543). Paternal suicide, as Landon experienced, is known to complicate normal developmental tasks, particularly in adolescents who rely on healthy idealization and identification of caregivers in order to differentiate and establish a sense of autonomy. In accord with that formulation, Tillman adds that

> The suicide of a family member, particularly a parent, often inflicts a moral injury on surviving family members . . . and for children and adolescents this may have a profound effect on the task of mourning and reestablishing a stable link to the moral order, a protective factor against suicide.
>
> (p. 563)

Landon's hospitalization occurred more than thirty years ago—long before the concept of moral injury was developed and applied by Tillman. While I would still initiate diagnosis and treatment with similar principles as described throughout the chapter, I would now include in therapy with Landon and in supervision the importance of discussing moral injury. I would spell out that moral injury occurred by the suicide first, and then by the multiple and multifarious levels of family secret keeping.

Naming the paternal suicide as a moral injury to Landon's developing self would initiate the discussion. I would then add that, for Landon, a sense of moral injury occurred on two major levels: the suicide of his father, obviously, and then the years of cover-up and obfuscation at the behest of his mother. Although secret keeping as such is not routinely thought of as morally injurious, the multiple levels at which it occurred for Landon derailed his thinking and led to severe depression. Following Tillman's clinical observations, I would ask Landon questions about how the demand to keep so much undercover complicated his sense of right and wrong.

"Suicide opens a door for the next generation. You don't want to put that burden on the back of your children or grandchildren," is an intervention long used by clinicians to help stop impulsive action as Landon threatened to do. It's not meant to be as heavy-handed or preachy as it may sound. Without calling out the moral injury per se, clinicians may have been inadvertently grasping for the moral injury concept Tillman fleshes out in her research to help curtail intergenerational trauma.

Now, I remind patients like Landon that by staying alive, they are breaking a noxious intergenerational pattern that could lead to the suicide of loved one years later. Good is actually being done even when the patient feels the worst and is convinced that life is not worth living: they are reestablishing a sense of moral order and ongoing hope for the family.

Tillman stresses that the therapist must be comfortable with their own aggression to survive the attacks, both conscious and unconscious, that derive from patients' unexpressed anger, guilt, and fantasies of hate and aggression. Moral injury is further complicated when the survivor of familial suicide does not know what led up to the "decision to end one's life . . . Survivors of parental suicide may develop a fantasy that the parent had wished for the child to die as well or was indifferent to the child's life or death" (p. 545). The secret keeping in Landon's family was morally injurious because truth was shut down, perhaps exacerbating unconscious fantasies that his own father may have wanted him to die and that his mother's needs were more important than his own.

The circumstances of the death and admonitions for the hermetically sealed secret keeping in this family, just as in other cases, will never be completely and precisely understood. Still, in treatment, I now underscore to patients like Landon that these hidden stories no longer need be kept, but the fact that they had to do so for so many years has led to burdens on the mind and body. No matter how painful, it is essential to share in treatment any thoughts, fantasies, and temptations to hurt oneself. I encourage patients to assume that anxiety will emerge when they attempt to do just this. In this way, we gently confront and give voice to the resistance we know from the start will be part of the process to shut down the open, healing dialogue we seek.

Another additional but related approach includes emphasizing that while we will never know what lies behind a loved one's decisions or within their thinking process, we all have thoughts and fantasies about why a person takes the actions they do. Therapy frees a patient to consider those facts and talk about them. The therapeutic task is not to dodge these questions but to welcome their emergence from the shadowy underground. When brought to the surface and faced, mental pain is diminished. To solidify the developmental achievement of ambivalent object relations, the therapist must also give explicit permission for the patient to tell us when they feel let down and disappointed with us—another goad in the process of facing down the injurious sealed lips of their past.

Conclusion

Secret keeping can have unanticipated but deleterious impact on the body and mind. Some pieces of personal history that are hiding in plain view frequently but surreptitiously metastasize to include admonitions, messages, and unspoken orders to stay silent. They may serve a protective psychological function for an individual who benefits from concealing information but places other human beings in an emotionally exhausting, complicit role. Sometimes, unwitting participants like caretakers or parents impinge on those dependent on them to sustain them emotionally or to unconsciously assist with emotional regulation. In the most egregious circumstances (e.g., incest, rape, abuse), the collusive alliance to stay silent augments damage exacted by the horrific event.

Those secrets associated with complicated bereavement, physical and psychological abuse, or severe family conflict have physical consequences in part because significant effort must be exerted to keep excruciating memories and psychological pain at bay. Feelings are excluded from awareness to preserve interpersonal attachments and allow a person to remain engaged in life. This kind of stress takes energy and eats away at the brain and body regardless of the kind of trauma that has occurred. The individual becomes inured to the defensive tendrils imposed by trying to live in two worlds at once. It's a life-zapping maneuver.

Emotional exhaustion born of the chronic stress of secret keeping has both physiological and psychological impact that must be explained to the patient, but only after the conditions of safety are met. Whether they are a suicidal risk or a highly functional troubled person, an effective therapist must first create the conditions that potentiate secure attachment. That way, early impingements can be recognized and, to some extent, reconfigured. The individual is then able to release their secrets and the pressures that encase them. In order to mend, the patient can begin to piece them together, into a conscious, consistent narrative that makes sense.

As we will see in the next chapter, splits in the psyche of some secret keepers are sometimes so profound that they are forced to live a double life. The consequence of sustained compartmentalization and this level of concealment takes us further into assessing the deleterious impact on mind and body and the pernicious aftereffects incurred to the individual or to loved ones who discover the cover-up.

Note

1 The late Dr. Irwin Rosen, psychotherapy maven and director of the Adult Psychotherapy Service at the Menninger Clinic for many years, advised younger colleagues promoted to similar roles that the new position came with risks and benefits. Potentially explosive situations and pieces of gossip about the lives of others in the clinic, community, and nation would be heard. There were more nuggets than one could imagine when accepting the job that had to be managed. The clinician had to find ways to cordon off this information overload and keep it to oneself; it was part of the new position to contain and to metabolize what was heard off the grid, so to speak. In essence, Rosen espoused a form of healthy dissociation (making use of the movable walls of the vertical split described in Chapter 1), and by his example demonstrated that it could be done admirably and successfully without excessive compromise to one's selfhood. He often highlighted his points with apt literary quotations that provided guidance and consolation simultaneously: "Don't secrete the secret. As Balzac put it, 'Memories beautify life, but only forgetting makes it bearable.'"

3   The Afterlife of a Double Life

All my life he had been in my corner, less an ancillary parent and more the big-brother type who introduced me to roller coasters, disco, and theater. So taking on "the powers," as the attorneys had put it when the duties of trustee were explained, was an easy call: Uncle Kirk had always been clear about his wishes, especially that I assume the role of administrative caretaker if he ever needed it. A few nights before all the lights went out, Uncle Kirk called in a rage.

I hadn't been sanguine ten years before when the well-meaning doctor told me that my uncle's fierce will to live would likely make him "a very long-term survivor" of the neurological disorder that now slowly whittled away at his once-facile intelligence and exuberant personality. Contorted by dueling sensations of reassurance and dread, I nonetheless managed to shrug off any intimation that the end was finally within sight. These days I toggled between feeling exhausted by the incessant demands of the tasks and feeling ashamed even to nurse private grudges, given all that we meant to each other.

Family lore touted that my uncle proudly conferred my nickname (and its unusual spelling), Kassy, at the hospital nursery. I was shaken when he revised history by blurting out early in his cognitive decline that the special sobriquet was actually the invention of Maisie Thomas, the expert seamstress in my grandfather's dry-cleaning plant. The apathetic tone with which Uncle Kirk rendered the revelation reflected the loss of another filter, not the unburdening of a guilty conscience.

Another step in the downward drift jolted me when he insisted that my grandmother, dead for more than two decades, had come into his room at the nursing home and eaten all his potato chips. Usually, it was easy to settle him or at least believe that he would respond to reassurances that his mother would soon return with more of his favorite snacks. I secured the collusion by asking the nursing staff at the facility to look in on him frequently and to monitor his confusion.

DOI: 10.4324/9781003471578-4

Instances of creeping demise piled up subtly over the decade but were remarkably consistent with the man I once knew. For this I counted myself lucky. There were some particularly good days when we watched his favorite movies from the 1940s, boisterously sang along, and spontaneously followed with choruses of his favorite show tunes of the period. Reminiscences of the campground where he and his best friend Leon went swimming in the 1930s; large, loud, animated family dinners during the post–World War II years; and travels with my late Aunt Grace in the 1950s and 1960s—these were all the data I needed to be certain that Uncle Kirk's memory of past events was intact.

The fury that spilled out now in what was to be our penultimate conversation went harum-scarum and frightened me. "After we got back from my doctor, Leon laid down the law. 'That's five bucks, Kirk,' he said, 'No more free rides. This car doesn't move unless you pay me!'" Uncle Kirk was bellowing. My attempt to appease him by promising to clarify the matter about the alleged rift with Leon, his closest friend since childhood, only exacerbated his frenzy. Wondering whether my uncle was becoming slightly paranoid or delusional about what his childhood friend intended, I offered to call Leon's daughter to make things right or repair any damage.

> Don't you dare . . . I'm done . . .Years of footing his bill . . .pulling him out of manholes and mischief . . . Now he charges me for a ride . . . I know where the bodies are buried. There are plenty of them!

Dumbfounded because he rarely grew agitated with me before this moment, I sensed disappointment and grief beneath Uncle Kirk's demand that I could not easily redress this time. My heart sank. Did this ache signal another layer of my personal loss, or was it emotion that I was also trying to contain and manage for my failing uncle? Without warning, Uncle Kirk's deteriorating mind momentarily cleared, puncturing my internal reverie, and he shouted a final order. "I insist you say none of this to anyone, Kassy! I will deal with Leon myself."

A spiral into total silence and toward death took another couple of months. Once as I stroked his forehead at the bedside in hospice, Uncle Kirk was able to utter, "Thank you, dear," but there was no semblance of conversation, let alone a word or two to fill the gap about what had transpired between him and Leon. I struggled against my proclivity to be curious and dismissed suggestions that my friends had made for years: "Stop trying to matchmake for your uncle. He's clearly gay!"

"Leon and Kirk can't take their eyes off each other when they're together. They speak silently like an old married couple."

"You're not picking up on any of his nonverbal cues. For an otherwise smart shrink, I have to say you're behind the eight ball on this one."

Dismissing my friends' observations with a barely audible "nah" and wrinkle of my brow, conversation ceased. I refused to acknowledge what was so evident to all with eyes to see.

Uncle Kirk and Leon had more going on than friendship, and likely had for decades, despite the appearance of being respectable family men of the late twentieth century. Their secret materialized only as I ruffled through personal effects discovered within dark walnut bookcases that Uncle Kirk had carefully purged years before dementia took hold. A couple of gay porn films, rail passes for two to distant cities, and an odd assortment of receipts and notes outlined the depth of a relationship that was now irrefutable.

Were these souvenirs that a telltale heart unconsciously forgot? Or treasured keepsakes sequestered privately for reminiscence? Did Uncle Kirk want me to know all along? Had Leon's moneygrubbing broken his heart? Was Leon's perplexing conduct a sign of his own battle with guilt or loss? Questions swirled. And at what cost? The wisp extinguished itself abruptly after the secret—one that should never have been kept between us—came out.

Surprising Illuminations

Have you ever also been caught totally off guard by a sudden revelation about someone you thought you know well? Were you bewildered because you sensed something inexplicable that you just couldn't put your finger on? The news may have had the paradoxical effect of bringing clarity while instantly raising tension to a boil. Perhaps you sensed a shift in your body— flushing face, racing heartbeat, rumbling tummy, trembling fingertips, or teetering legs. After you didn't faint and nausea didn't send you racing toward the bathroom, you may have noticed how quickly your mind settled into the adaptive but nebulous process of digesting the information.

You may have felt something like my patient Michael did after his parents told him at age fifteen that his father had been married before and he had two half-siblings whom he had never met. Now an adult who runs his own plumbing business, he has gained perspective. "Suddenly what was so botched up in my family made sense," he said. "A puzzle fit together. At first, I was furious that they kept me in the dark! But then I felt a lot of stress settle and I started to do better in school." Many of us have noticed feelings of lucidity and decreased anxiety when a veil is peeled back and a fuller picture of an individual or our family background comes into clearer view.

It's easy to dismiss these observations because they can often happen quickly, seemingly randomly, almost like a bit of hocus-pocus. In this chapter, we deepen our perspective on the psychological and physical effects

of secret keeping on the body. So that we don't give short shrift when these mysterious happenstances occur, I present additional observations from the fields of medicine, neuropsychoanalysis, bereavement and grief research, and cognitive psychology. Revelations may temporarily blindside us but ultimately prove illuminating. As ever, the point is not to avoid having secrets—because that is impossible—but to emphasize the multiple ways that they impact us and those we love and to provide some tactics for dealing with them healthfully.

Clinical observation and cognitive research suggest that secret keeping may affect the brain as well as influence long-term physical and emotional well-being. It's another porthole that can help us reframe what we divulge to others, what we keep to ourselves, and how we go about sorting through those perplexing and ambiguous aftereffects that occur in life.

As with my Uncle Kirk and his lover, Leon, learning unforeseen facts about another person's life after they die is common, particularly for those charged with sifting through personal belongings or executing an estate. As psychoanalysts have also found, we all have unconscious wishes to gather some keys, bits of logic, or pieces of history that can, as my patient Michael ruefully confided, make one's life circumstances finally make sense. The fulfillment of even the most sought-after yearning to understand more about those we love is only ever partial and, in the case of a revealed secret, will usually prompt more questions than it answers.

Often this information is exciting to learn: the once ineffable takes on a human face! Witness the multimillion business of genealogy research and genetic testing that uncover roots in generations long departed. More is at stake psychologically than learning about one's biological lineage and family tree. News items abound detailing life histories rewritten for those who undertake this journey only to find out their parentage was decidedly different than they were led to believe.[1]

What is unearthed can prove emotionally taxing and time-consuming because it requires considerable revision in our mind of family members whom we thought we knew, and the revelation may usher in a delayed or complicated mourning process. It takes on a particularly troublesome valence for those individuals who are cut off from the usual supports that accompany loss. Some secrets—a miscarriage, abortion, imprisoned family member, severe financial reversal—may be deemed too shameful to speak about openly. Conversations with friends that could be sustaining don't happen. One bears one's loss alone; the toll on relationships is silent. This process—disenfranchised grief—may very well have influenced Leon's behaviors that seemed so crass and inscrutable at the time. The nature of his relationship with my uncle was such that he also bore witness to Uncle Kirk's incremental decline but had no one with whom he could safely speak, given their secrecy.

Later in the chapter, I provide a heartrending cinematic example of disenfranchised grief to amplify the concept a bit more. Suffice to say once again how the safe space of psychodynamic psychotherapy or psychoanalysis may play a healing role for anyone whose life turns upside down after an unexpected illumination. Somatic illness and body reactivity may attenuate when otherwise unspeakable losses and secrets can be openly discussed and sufficiently worked through. I conclude with some additional thoughts gleaned from cognitive research about how the act of writing and other creative forms of meaning making may be additional avenues to process secrets.

What Comes to Life after Death?

Novelists and screenwriters make their livelihood by portraying individuals whose lives are unexpectedly illuminated when a secret is revealed, particularly after death. In *The Bridges of Madison County*, the protagonist Francesca Johnson leaves behind a letter and some artifacts for her son and daughter to find after she dies: she wants her children to know she had a great love in her life—besides her husband. She also directs them to have her ashes cremated and spread near her lover's instead of burying her next to their father, which initially mortifies her children when they read her will. During her lifetime, Francesca told no one about her brief affair with photographer Robert Kincaid, ostensibly because she did not wish to disturb the security of her husband and children, whom she also loved. I always wondered why this novel (which was also made into a highly successful, Oscar-nominated film starring Meryl Streep and Clint Eastwood) was an international bestseller, appealing to millions of people, particularly women.

In part, this story satisfies our unconscious wish to set the record straight about beloved figures, such as mothers, whom we can only ever know partially and imperfectly. The idea of a matriarch who relinquishes her own passions for her husband and children has been an irresistible subject in the arts for centuries, appealing not only to our imagination but also to our infantile need for protection and fusion with an unassailable, idealizable parent.

I have also felt that a particular allure of *The Bridges of Madison County* is the twist it gives to the unconscious quest to know more about one's parent—and its implicit encouragement to embrace affirming and unanticipated possibilities in the present moment. Permission is granted from the grave by Francesca to her adult children: they should live their lives on their own terms, just as she had. Revealing her love affair in the discovered notebooks and photographs tacitly encourages her son and daughter to pursue their own dreams, even if fleeting or painful. In a final letter explaining the conflict she faced in choosing between her love for Robert and her family, Francesca writes, "I only wish that someday you each might have what I experienced; however, I'm beginning to think that's not likely" (Waller, 1992, p. 154).

Liberation so awakened is palpable in the text. After both adult children metabolize the discombobulating information they just learned about their mother, they speak to how their bodies feel lighter, calmer, and stronger. They fall silent, take deep breaths, wipe away tears and beads of perspiration, and gently whisper to each other what they take for granted in their current lives; in the kitchen where their mother's four-day affair unfolded, they begin to cogitate about what can still change. Finally, they wash down their reactions with a sip of her brandy, an implicit toast to the past and a nod to an imagined future.

Eventually deciding to go public with the story about Francesca and Robert's love affair with the help of the fictional narrator, a journalist, the siblings radiate warmth and empathy with details of the poignant tale that they insist will enlighten their fellow human beings. The background figure of the journalist, carefully listening and obviously moved by the details, assumes the role of witness. In a way, the narrator acts as therapist for the siblings, who need to work through this revised picture of their mother and family history. This satisfies another less conscious but very human desire to have time and space to absorb a mother's canny and yearned-for "gift from the crypt"—a gentle prod to her surviving children so that they might embrace their one and only life with less self-deception and more courage.

Self-Regulatory Depletion: Another Cost of Concealment

Over the years, I have seen patients improve considerably—with their eating disorders, addictions, anxiety, and even cognitive symptoms—after they acknowledge facts that have been hitherto hidden, but in plain view. I've also been struck by how often individuals begin to think clearer and do better in school or at their jobs when previous deceptions or secrets in one's family of origin come out from the shadows and into the open.

After the discovery of Uncle Kirk's secret life, I began to wonder whether long-term, self-imposed concealment of essential facts about one's identity might be one factor leading to cognitive, behavioral, or medical decline. Digging into cognitive and social psychology research yielded some astonishing and unexpected results. In 2014, researchers Clayton Critcher and M. J. Ferguson found that that there are measurable costs to keeping information concealed even in experimental situations where the environment is controlled. In what psychologists call "self-regulatory depletion," intellectual acuity, physical stamina, and executive function all drop when one is trying to avoid giving away information.

If the taboo was detected during the experiment, speech was spontaneously modified for content to keep up the ruse. Concealment produces physical and emotional depletion even when there is no need to monitor speech, suggesting that secret keeping may prevent people from optimal cognitive performance in many kinds of situations. Indeed, secret keepers perform 17 percent worse than controls on spatial intelligence tests—a fact that those of us who keep secrets for a living need to remember!

The keeper of secrets must have the capacity to switch back and forth between different mental states or mindsets quickly. Consider this endearing example: a parent privately muses on the special birthday gift they picked for their child's birthday—something they know the child doesn't expect but will be thrilled to receive. The child walks into the room, disrupting the fantasy. The parent must quickly switch gears. Focus turns to the child. Restraint prevails. The wily adult can push the surprise to the side and not blurt out a clue. Several brain regions have done their job perfectly in milliseconds and the change in mindset isn't noticed. This aspect of executive functioning, however, requires self-regulation that carries psychic costs that add up over a day (Hamilton, Vohs, Sellier, & Meyvis, 2011; Maranges & Baumeister, 2016). Experiments demonstrate that switching mindsets exhausts self-regulatory resources, leading to failure in self-control, negative moods, and ultimately self-regulatory collapse.

Functional neuroimaging links this kind of self-regulatory depletion to increased amygdala activity, reduced functional connectivity, and decoupling between the left amygdala and ventromedial prefrontal cortex, particularly if the stimulus is perceived as negative or conflictual (Heatherton & Wagner, 2011; Wagner & Heatherton, 2013). Continuous monitoring—as is needed to keep a secret—can make for a particularly stressful situation requiring unconscious effort to regulate emotion, thoughts, and behaviors. Intuitively, we know this fact because we've been in situations where we've had to keep our lips sealed. It takes willpower and energy to bat away something that we know cannot or should not be disclosed. The more we try and stop it, the more it seems to bubble to the tip of consciousness. We try to avoid these encounters that are baffling and frustrating. Now, science is beginning to pin down precisely what happens and the neurocircuitry involved at the brain level when we expend energy for such precisely titrated self-regulation. Evidence continues to mount that smoking, drinking alcohol, taking drugs, and excessive eating result from self-regulatory failures processed in the prefrontal regions (Sayette & Creswell, 2016; Wagner & Heatherton, 2013, 2015).

Given these forays into the contemporary cognitive psychology and neurology literature, it seems increasingly plausible to me that secrets accumulated over the course of a lifetime can have a decidedly negative impact on the brain. Are there other stories like my uncle's that, even if considered circumstantial, can provide additional plausible evidence? Genetic factors, medical illnesses, and biological markers yet to be discovered are the linchpins underlying cognitive decline and dementia in contemporary medicine. I initially considered my question to be the fanciful wish of a niece trying to make some sense of her Uncle Kirk's sudden deterioration and the utterly complex, yet only partially known, etiologies of dementia. Then, I stumbled upon a fascinating book on healthy aging that offered a corroborating and unexpected point of view.

Leaks and Confessions of Elderly Patients in Psychotherapy

Esteemed psychoanalyst and educator Danielle Quinodoz's book *Growing Old: A Journey of Self-Discovery* (2009) is a resource for remaining vital in one's later years. As part of her long career in mental health treatment, teaching, and writing, Dr. Quinodoz consulted with nursing homes in her native Switzerland for decades. There she taught and supervised the younger generations of psychotherapists who were helping elderly residential patients review the scope of their lives, gain mastery over existential concerns and fear of death, and stay as creative and actively involved in living as they could. Her synthesis is a guide for anyone who hopes for an abundant harvest during one's senior years, brimming as it is with many patient examples and specific advice.

Tucked in the pages was one astute observation I never expected to see. Over the years of treating literally hundreds of nursing home patients, Dr. Quinodoz and her younger colleagues were struck by how many disclosed a riveting part of their personal history in therapy that they never dared share with anyone else. These included stories of adoption, parental abandonment, sexual abuse, death of a sibling or child, abortion, miscarriage, and disappointment in or betrayal by a loved one. Resentments lingered. Psychosomatic illnesses magnified. Regrets and guilt accumulated. The storyteller often wept.

Prior to dying or descending into the final stage of dementia, these patients unburdened themselves by revealing their conflicts and feelings to their therapist. As memory closes its door, the therapist serves as witness. And after the highly personal, historical detail was told, some patients, like my Uncle Kirk, no longer communicated meaningfully with any staff or family member. It was as if the scribe in the form of the therapist appeared just in time, before all the lights went out.

These revelations—the secret sharing and the cessation of further communication at the end of life—led Dr. Quinodoz to suspect that mental decline has a psychological function. Sometimes, it occurs to stave off mourning and anxiety about death, while downplaying particular facets about oneself that one would like to disown or disavow. Protecting one's family or friends may be one advantage, but there are health and relationship consequences of mental decline. By sidestepping regret or dodging remorse, the last stage of life for an elderly person is impoverished. What is felt as shameful or destructive remains hidden and cannot be processed.

Most of us have aspects of our identity that we prefer to keep to ourselves and can empathize with those who choose to avoid disclosure on account of social taboo. In today's world, a closeted sexual orientation may seem like a relic of the past, but Uncle Kirk and Leon struggled with the stigma attached to homosexual relationships because they grew up in the United States during the Second World War. Even as society made significant advances in accepting gay relationships over the course of their lives, both men kept their relationship under wraps for personal, private reasons, about which we can only speculate. Historical, cultural, religious, and family context must always be taken into consideration when it comes to the secrets one keeps or reveals.

We all grapple at times with the moral complexities around secrets. At times, can keeping a secret be a moral failing? What might be the impact on others if we hold, or reveal, a secret? How might we rationalize or feign ignorance of someone else's emotional plight or conflict? I come back to this in Chapter 6, but for now suffice to say that both—the person with the secret to keep, and an individual who would prefer that they never heard it—have important questions to sort through as evidence mounts about the emotional and physical consequences of secret keeping. These are the additional unanticipated and deleterious aftereffects of knowing what you are not supposed to know and feeling what you are not supposed to feel—to use Bowlby's turn of phrase.

Dr. Quinodoz's clinical material raises another thorny question that we clinicians cannot fully answer in the present, but it primes us to always keep our ears open and minds alert to the ineffable: Does keeping a secret for years eat its way into an individual's soul? Should clinicians be listening for secrets as an additional factor affecting physical, emotional, and neurological well-being? The following tales are chilling examples of mindboggling whole-body perplexities.

Other Double Lives

At the time of diagnosis of a malignant brain tumor, journalist Caroline Knapp's father confessed to his wife that he had an ongoing extramarital affair that had supposedly ended ten years prior. In her memoir, *Drinking: A Love Story* (1996), Knapp describes this death bed confession and the fallout for her family. Her father, a prominent Boston psychoanalyst, offered a number of reasons for his betrayal and for keeping it hushed up until he faced death. For one thing, the location of the cancer crossed the midline of his brain, involving both his left and right cortex. Essentially, the tumor split him in two.

For Dr. Knapp, the brain tumor represented an unresolved psychosomatic conflict, a bifurcated sense of himself as father, husband, and psychiatrist as well as his clandestine life with the other woman. He hinted at other issues of personal avoidance on which he had gained perspective and offered advice to his daughter, then in the throes of severe alcoholism. Caroline Knapp eventually took it to heart. He incisively confronted a façade that he believed was ruining her life: "There is a split with you, and you *must* deal with it. You *must*," he entreated (p. 201; italics in original).

Dramatic stories that are richly described in memoir and biography may still be easily pushed to the side because we can't yet make an absolute link between the secret and a disorder of magnitude. Their psychosomatic angle sounds like so much fantasy. Still, when we pause to listen for them or begin to scope them out, we start to wonder about the residual effect of secret keeping on the body. Frequently, concealment encompasses issues of trauma, grief, suicide, and loss. With afflictions such as dementia, brain tumor, addiction, and sudden onset or perpetuation of physical disease, a split in the psyche may be a contributing factor.

A colleague of mine supervised a young professional woman in her clinical practice, who worked incessantly hard but whose disorganization and inability to cooperate with others caused problems in the office (Frankfeldt, 2019). When she met with this student in supervision, the psychoanalyst, Valerie Frankfeldt of New York City, felt herself becoming sad and perplexed. When the student unexpectedly withdrew from work due to a severe back injury and ended her practicum, she was surprised at the relief she felt. Uncharacteristically, over the months, she continued to puzzle about how the student's departure mysteriously lifted weight off her own back even as she remained curious about how the student was doing.

Two years later, Dr. Frankfeldt was contacted by this student, who revealed that her mother had committed suicide just before she began her placement. Dr. Frankfeldt then understood both the reason for the student's behavior and her own physical reactivity when trying to supervise her. Although the student did not intend to keep her mother's suicide a secret, thereby throwing everyone in the office into turmoil, unable to support her, she had managed to cordon off her loss through unrelenting activity—that is, until her injury forced her to quit and take time to mourn.

By mechanisms still only partially understood by science, Dr. Frankfeldt sensed the sadness surrounding the mother's death that her student had temporarily and successfully walled off and deposited into her. What was disavowed by the student had taken up residence in my colleague's psyche, causing disquieting splits in consciousness for each. The student was unable or simply reluctant to acknowledge and assimilate the effects of her mother's suicide at the time of her placement. Experience enabled Dr. Frankenfeldt to address her own disparate sense of self at that time: "Something is happening inside me when I sit with this person that just isn't me, and I don't understand yet. I need to think about it." In this way, she was able to more fully comprehend and integrate when additional information revealed itself.

Over her years of clinical practice, Dr. Frankenfeldt has come to trust her instincts, and she urges other therapists to do likewise because it deepens the psychotherapeutic experience. Noting that the perplexity created by these sensations can be unnerving when first encountered—and therefore dismissed—she nonetheless has learned that physical sensations (hunger, nausea, tightness in the chest, and changing heart rate) and behavioral symptoms (derealization, depersonalization, and changes in body image) offer essential data about a patient's subjectivity and emotional experience. Dr. Frankfeldt is one of a key group of contemporary psychoanalysts[2] whose written work I cite throughout the book as further evidence of how the body simultaneously holds and offers up information about the patient that is unattainable otherwise and thus tends to remain silent, sequestered, and secret unless the therapist welcomes it into the dialogue.

Disenfranchised Grief

The common thread linking Leon, Dr. Knapp's mistress, Dr. Frankfeldt's student, and even some of Dr. Quinodoz's patients who bore their unspeakable losses silently is what psychologists call disenfranchised grief (Attig, 2004; Doka, 1999, 2002). When grief is experienced by someone who is not in a position to publicly acknowledge their loss, it becomes impossible for them to mourn and to move forward into life. Support systems that come to the aid of mourners, such as friends or spiritual community, are not usually available to those who have harbored relationships that must be disavowed in society or who have gone through something stigmatizing, like the suicide of a loved one.

When we consider the cost of secret keeping for whatever reason, we inevitably ignore those impacted who are left to mourn by themselves because their loss is not perceived. Carolyn Knapp's memoir never says another word about her father's mistress, who was left to weather the loss of a long-term love on her own. Perhaps involvement in a secret touches off a tad of schadenfreude, especially if we know and care about those impacted by the secret keeping. We may not say it out loud, but judgment does cross our mind: "They did it to themselves. They deserve their misery so let them wallow in it."

A compelling cinematic example of disenfranchised grief won the Academy Award for Best Foreign Film in 2018. In the Chilean film *A Fantastic Woman* (Lelio & Maza, 2017), the main character, Marina, is a transgender woman who lives in Santiago with her male lover, Orlando. After his sudden death, Marina is forbidden to attend his funeral, to take ownership of their dog Diabla or any material possessions, or to continue living temporarily in their apartment. In effect, her lover's surviving family totally and cruelly denies their relationship, both publicly and personally. While the relationship of Marina and Orlando was not itself a secret, his survivors want to keep their affair as quiet as possible in the town. As we empathize with the main character, whose grief is totally minimized and discounted, moviegoers are left to imagine for ourselves the shame accompanying the slights of the deceased's family members.

Disenfranchised grief comes in many forms, and now we see it being studied for its impact on professional burnout in particular (Lathrop, 2017). Acknowledging loss and anticipating the subtleties of burnout are recommended, but it's often difficult to be in touch with our grief and bodily and psychic reactivity as they happen. So much emotional exhaustion, cumulative losses, and sense of falling short can come with a job. The accompanying pain feels unacceptable. Burnout creeps in clandestinely, eventually shattering the obliviousness of its victim. Physicians, teachers, ministers, caregivers of the elderly, and palliative care providers are some of the professionals that are especially afflicted, because they are entrusted with mounds of confidential information and the pile up of unexpressed grief.

Given the ubiquity of disenfranchised grief, we all likely harbor elements of it that we take for granted or ignore until it is brought to awareness. Short of entering psychotherapy, what steps can an individual take to reconcile the innumerable losses and transitions that build up over the years and burrow into the psyche and body? Throughout the book, I've tried to include helpful guidelines and practical tips for anyone holding a vexing secret as well as for those who share their confidence—namely, those individuals who are good at holding private information for loved ones and friends or who come to the task because of their role in a professional relationship. Here's one of those tips.

Writing: Another Resource for the Secret Keeper

In many wisdom traditions, writing is a spiritual practice. In her book *Writing Down the Bones* (1986), poet and educator Natalie Goldberg reminds us of that and passes on advice for the personal value of writing in human predicaments. She lyrically describes the value of writing confirmed by psychological research, cited later in the chapter. When it comes to processing human anguish, Goldberg observes:

> Writing is the act of burning through the fog in your brain. . . . . Writing is not therapy, though it may have a therapeutic effect . . . You write

through your pain, and even your suffering must be written out and let go of . . . Writing gives you a great opportunity to swim through to freedom . . .Writing has tremendous energy.

(pp. 148, 190–191)

Is it possible that writing down one's secrets is another way of metabolizing the emotional impact? Might writing positively influence health outcomes and enhance emotional reserves? With situations such as disenfranchised grief, bitter memories, and betrayal, and emotions such as anger, guilt, and shame, the page offers safe reservoir, facilitating relief from anguish and ensuring privacy. While a substitute for neither psychotherapy nor a non-judgmental, insightful confidant, elucidating a nugget or "the bone" of the story may help secret keepers manage the invisible burden. Complicated pining, congeries of memories, and nostalgia tinged with regret must otherwise be stored behind sealed lips.

During the COVID-19 pandemic, psychoanalyst and author Kerry Malawista invited experienced psychodynamic psychotherapists and psychoanalysts and professional writers to join her in providing small group workshops for frontline responders (Malawista, 2021 a, b). The resource offered was a writing intervention. Participants were encouraged to talk about what they wrote, but first they had to write. The volunteer professionals who led the groups stayed focused on the material the members produced. While the intervention had some elements of "the talking cure," talking was not the primary mode of therapeutic action.

By putting words on paper to gain self-awareness and reveal the manifold stressors they had already experienced and were living through, emergency personnel, administrators, physicians, nurses, firemen, and law enforcement officers were given a tool to reshape and begin to process what they witnessed. A professional writer, a mental health professional, and other group members helped shape and refine the poems, short essays, and stories that flowed from the pens and keypads of the first responders in their small group. As vulnerabilities and moving incidents were tearfully recounted, a sense of safety grew. People who thought they had no capacity to turn a phrase learned that they could do so and were often quite good at it, promoting a sense of mastery of a new skill and resilience in the face of significant psychological turmoil.

In an interview with the *Baltimore Sun*, Dr. Malawista (2021a) further explained the rationale behind The Things They Carry Project:

Writing enables us to step back and to reflect on trauma and loss. It's healing to create a narrative of what has happened to us. . . I've come to understand that writing transforms pain, anxiety, dread, and from disjointed images into reimagined images that one can begin to bear.

In fact, a robust store of psychological literature supports the use of writing to address many life circumstances, especially trauma and loss. I've wondered about its applicability to those *who believe they must keep their secret only to themselves.* These are the silently carried burdens that engender the harmful personal, psychological, and health impacts described throughout this book.

To sort out whether writing about personally upsetting experiences could be useful, psychologist James Pennebaker and colleagues conducted research with college students who had experienced a trauma (Pennebaker, 1989, 1993; Pennebaker & Beal, 1986; Pennebaker & Chung, 2007; Pennebaker & Smyth, 2016; Pennebaker & Susman, 1988). In a series of papers beginning in the 1980s, the psychologists compared those asked to write about their experience (usually for fifteen to thirty minutes on three to five consecutive days) to control groups who did not.

Consistently, those who wrote had improved health outcomes compared to the controls. Pennebaker concluded that writing is linked to improvement because the process itself is doing something more than serving as a catharsis. The construction of a coherent story with the expression of emotion, particularly negative emotion, is what makes writing a therapeutic experience.

In contrast to Malawista's writing groups, the students kept their journals and notebooks completely private. Bypassing a sense of shame or embarrassment may be key to the personal impact of Pennebaker's intervention, but similar brain-based mechanisms are ultimately at work for anyone who decides to put this research to use in their life. Cooling down the sympathetic nervous system, increasing prefrontal activation, and downregulating the amygdala and autonomic nervous system may be key facilitators of improved body-mind synergy for the secret keeper who writes down what they cannot share.

While no absolute conclusions can yet be drawn, the scientific evidence about the value of writing continues to expand and is suggestive of possible value for anyone with baggage to unpack. This is why I sometimes advise patients with a secret to hold to write down "just the bone"—or bullet points of what they carry in between sessions even when they tell me they aren't natural writers. Talent is not what matters. The benefit is derived simply from scaffolding one's narrative and simultaneously discharging the neurobiological load. The individual must then decide whether it is better to rip up their notes or locate a secure place to store them.

How many novelists, screenwriters, and nonfiction writers have shared secrets in their personal lives by documenting them in the transformed narrative of a novel, poem, memoir, or biography? One must be intentional, of course, about storing a story. The fictitious Francesca Johnson *wanted* her children to discover her letter in their heirloom cedar chest. Those who don't want to be discovered should bury the key.

A Little Bit More about Michael and Me

During Michael's three years of twice-weekly individual psychotherapy, I tried to pry open any stored-away reactions that he had about finding out about his half-siblings in his adolescence. While the boys all met each other on several occasions, they had no regular contact in adulthood. They knew about each other's families but never chose to visit or get close.

Michael's experience dramatically contrasted with jubilant encounters we read about in the press when people discover lost relatives. A new phase of life appears to be ushered in for some who can claim a previously unknown family member that expands their circle. As Michael's therapist, I was concerned that he was missing out on this potential opportunity by walling off a slew of resentments and anger toward his parents and unconscious competitive and embarrassing feelings toward his older half-brothers.

When Michael spoke about any member of his adult family, I took it as an opening to say that he had not mentioned his half siblings for some time. They were part of his family too, I repeated. Why was he choosing to ignore this fact that was known to all? Were important memories or affects being defensively avoided?

Michael's answer was always the same. He said,

> Look, Dr. Z., it's like I told you before. Learning about my brothers when I was a teenager did have an impact, but I don't feel a sense of connection to them now. It's really all right. I think you think I am holding something back from you, but I'm not. I came to therapy for you to help me be more assertive toward my wife and stand up for son. That's what's helping.

I wondered whether Michael's passivity with his wife reflected his early experience of being a passive receptacle for information about his brothers that was hurtful and bewildering. I continued to attend to cues and to nudge him to connect elements of his conflicts when it seemed relevant.

Eventually, Michael called me out for importuning! He said,

> Let it go already. I don't need to talk about the brothers. Do you really think that writing—or even dictating my thoughts into my cell phone— is something a busy plumber is going to do? It's enough to make it here twice weekly for therapy. You get on my nerves whenever you bring this fact of my life up and seem to expect me to do something with it.

Michael made a valid point. I was glad to hear him speak his truth clearly and stand up for his perspective. Sometimes revealed secrets don't have the and cause unbearable loneliness. Because of the secrets we keep, we all likely harbor more disenfranchised grief than we are consciously aware of at any given moment. Attuning to its depleting forces may help us avoid burnout and cynicism.

It is impossible to predict what the impact of a newly revealed secret will be for any individual, so it's important to keep in mind that research offers some practical tools and wisdom that can help lift the emotional fog and inner turbulence created by the inevitable shifts, adjustments, and losses caused when something shocking comes to light. This emotional pain arrives as unpredictable waves for anyone who must readjust their picture of someone held dear. Talking with a trusted person and writing about the experience promote a working-through of this new and more complete image. The revised but fuller perspective is ultimately relieving and healing, which I appreciate all the more as I consider my discoveries about my beloved Uncle Kirk.

Notes

1 Journalist Libby Copeland's book *The Lost Family: How DNA Testing Is Upending Who We Are* (2020) is based on interviews of individuals who learned about their genetic parents from relative matching of companies like Ancestry and 23andMe. Secrets long withheld—what Copeland calls unexpected truths—have the power to significantly change family dynamics and reshape individual identities. One woman who discovered that her biological father was not the man who raised her, told Copeland that she "was devastated that I wasn't who I thought I was. I was made by a stranger." The popular PBS television series *Finding Your Roots*, produced by renowned Harvard professor Henry Louis Gates, delights audiences and enlightens its famous guests by probing their genealogical backgrounds. Advertised to educate Americans about the diverse histories and cultures that shape our common humanity by bringing to light complex and often hidden genetic family trees, guests invariably discover new facts and withheld secrets buried within their own families. Combining cutting-edge DNA research, the tools of a master historian, and a finely honed capacity for empathy, Gates assists his guests in processing the newly unearthed information, usually to their amazement. The recipients often say in the program that they will need to continue to further distill the new facts, attesting to their intuitive understanding that modification and remolding of the sense of self begins instantaneously but will take time to unpack. The family heritage and secrets may no longer be "dangerous" but are no less revealing, and the popularity of the show resides in part with the audience's identification that the subject is "one of us" who is able to withstand and grow from the solved mystery they came forward to share.

2 Unconscious communication between human beings is ubiquitous. Science is quickly advancing to offer different points of view on how this occurs. For example, based on her decades of research on multiple code theory, psychologist and psychoanalyst Wilma Bucci (1997, 2008, 2011a, b, 2018) found that unconscious emotional communication can be demonstrated at the brain level by fMRI and TMS studies in mammals and humans. Body movements, facial

expression, gestures, and vocal tone are e[...]
between giver and receiver instantaneou[...]
affective core that shape our interactions [...]
mate. Because human beings share neur[...]
ence as *uncanny* or *mystical* are actual w[...]
attuned neurological systems between ou[...]
dynamics, quantum mechanics, and matl[...]
at the boundary of interpersonal relations[...]
appreciate the complexity of unconscious [...]
pist that occurs within microseconds (Gi[...]
2008, 2011, 2017, 2018; Marks-Tarlow, 2[...]
1990; Shapiro & Marks-Tarlow, 2021).[...]
may also be understood as one of many in[...]
ized "into messy entanglements between s[...]
p. 114) that involve multiple, circular fee[...]
influences. Based on the evolving neurosci[...]
another "messy entanglement" involvin[...]
loops registered by mind and body.

**4 D[...]
ar[...]**

"My fath[...]
The pat[...]
months be[...]
office the [...]
A sixty[...]
interviews [...]
enhanced [...]
that psyc[...]
and adapt[...]
behind, h[...]
Our th[...]
analysis a[...]
seemingly [...]
est and h[...]
I looke[...]
she used [...]
feedback [...]
relaxing, [...]
relayed h[...]
recent de[...]
thesized t[...]
Consid[...]
the amia[...]
and chur[...]
expected [...]
meticulo[...]
A dow[...]
pull up t[...]
I tell yo[...]
stomach.

DOI: 10.43[...]

Whoosh! Not a moment to collect my thoughts. Dr. Dunn hit me with a wall of angry accusations about her father, stomping back and forth repeatedly from my desk to the couch, bellowing. She didn't pause to take a breath.

I hate him! Liar! No gentleman . . . I'm spitting fire . . . a poser! I couldn't believe my own eyes. I didn't want to get out of bed this morning, but Ollie insisted that I keep my therapy appointment. I feel as if I am unraveling. There's no balm a therapist can provide! What can be done when you find something like this out about someone you loved and trusted your entire life?

Totally upended by this outpouring of raw emotion, I found it impossible to follow her storyline. Helplessness surged. I wanted to flee. I wondered whether anyone in the next office heard her blast and might come running to my assistance.

Suddenly a piece of sage advice from discussions with colleagues early in my career made its way to consciousness like a welcome apparition. *Kassy, sometimes all you can do in a tempest is sit still in your chair. Take in what you can. Wait it out. If a patient's boomeranging gets under your skin and you flush or shed tears, that's human. It takes time to weather an onslaught.*[1]

I glanced at my bookshelf and favorite paintings apprehensively; they helped me withstand the barrage and tune in to the sense of mortification that underlay the patient's torrent. Over the weekend, Dr. Dunn and her spouse Ollie found memorabilia of parents and grandparents squirreled away in the family's vacation home. Precisely what unknown facts were now provoking vexation and anguish?

Gradually, Dr. Dunn simmered and plopped down on the couch, muttering under her breath. "Bastard! I still can't believe it! My own father—a pornographer!"

My own throat tightened. I could feel my stomach churn. Were my body signals alerting me to Dr. Dunn's anger that covered foreboding or deeper hurt and disappointment? How could I know whether these physical sensations belonged to her or to me? Apprehensive but curious, I decided to try to slow us both down.

I said, "It sounds excruciating. You were caught off guard and disgusted. Nasty nauseous aftermath! Can you tell me more about how you made the discovery?"

She elaborated. "I plunged my hands behind the 1970s cedar paneled wall in the den. We were ripping it out for the remodel. We found a huge stash of obscene pictures that Dad signed. I knew he liked to doodle but not draw nude models! I can't believe Ollie roared with amusement. It was obvious I was furious.

All four generations of our family vacationed in that two-story cabin on the lake near Wenatchee. What was I thinking? We started our update to get a better price before putting the place on the market. What we found makes my head spin and I want to retch."

I pointed out that the nude pictures she found did not make her father a pornographer; he wasn't selling vulgar images. I said I understood that this new information would take time to emotionally sort out. Pulling together threads from what I had heard so far led me to speculate that Dr. Dunn was sensing and seeing more than she could have ever anticipated when she began the staggering process of sorting through decades of her family's accumulated belongings. The chiaroscuros she found would take time to integrate into the internal image of her father. I asked her to continue her associations.

Dr. Dunn curled up on the couch, hugged a pillow, closed her eyes, and suddenly seemed to be a younger version of herself. She whimpered as she looked backward in time, and her thoughts unreeled. She confessed that she had made a second discovery over the weekend when she and Ollie happened upon the pictures.

> Along with the drawings we found other images in dusty cardboard boxes. Lots! Who would have thought? Maybe grandpa's lewd post-cards? A 1909 profile of a woman in a bustier with huge boobs and hips posing as if she was trying to touch a star? Cutouts of models drawn in their undies from old Sears Roebuck catalogues. A male boxer in black tights and undershirt with serious biceps threw me though. A camera obscura of turn-ons for my grandparents? The image unlocked a whole new flavor in my memory vault. Ugh. Dousing Christmas sand tarts with egg whites and cinnamon sugar like we did at our family's holiday baking parties will never feel the same.

Our talking together appeared to open a space for reflection and curi-osity. Equanimity was gaining ground. Her jovial manner momentarily reclaimed, Dr. Dunn proceeded to turn the tables on me and the psycho-therapy process. She blurted out a question and then answered it for her-self with new and important personal details.

"Is this what you people call unearthing 'multigenerational phantoms' or 'intergenerational ghosts'? I don't think I mean that as sarcastically as it sounds."

I paused. Dr. Dunn moistened her lips. She seemed to be shaking. I reminded her that therapy was a safe space to work through scary issues and that anger often shrouds anxiety. Her image of a little girl with Christ-mas cookies was poignant but tinged with animosity.

I inquired, "What else might be coming to mind about your past?"

> It's just that I've seen so much of bodies. At the women's prison where I did part time outpatient work, the collection of gadgets was astounding. People do weird stuff to get off. I kept a shoebox full of the screws, bolts, and hammerheads that I removed from the women's private parts in my garage for years. Who sneaks this stuff in? Extracting a tiny marble out of an old lady's ear and finding that she could then hear and wanted to dish her erotic experiences to me still gets top prize.

I murmured softly to let the patient know I was with her and grasping the intensity of her recollections and emotions. She had just let me in on her own secret collection and needed the refuge of the therapeutic space to gain perspective.

Dr. Dunn continued, widening the frame:

> The cabin's attic and closets were chock-full of stuff! Sets of Kodachrome slides that Dad must have picked up at the Moulin Rouge during their first European holiday were all thrown together in fraying manila envelopes. I bet Mom discovered them after he died. I suspect she was in on the gag. The full frontal black and white Polaroids of her and Auntie Este settled that question. I am going to save an 8 mm clip of mom jiggling her butt going up the steps at the Vatican. Dad must have filmed it himself. My playful, irreverent mother—I miss her. Other than that, it's all going up in smoke tonight over hot cider! We finally have use for that hideous cast iron fireplace insert they bought.

The appointment was coming to an end. I did not want her to feel alone or embarrassed. Much had been shared about the family secrets discovered during uncluttering that was new and unexpected and needed time to process.

I suggested, "Have you thought of waiting a bit? You don't have to chuck everything in the fire until you are ready."

She surprised me by concluding the session with a new angle on an old story she had spoken about several times before. It was playful this time.

"I know I've mentioned the professional junket we took to Fukuoka in 1989 but I never told you this one.

While I was in class with the other physicians, Ollie went to the train station to tour with the spouses. They discovered a slew of men's magazines loaded with pictures of bare feet and ankles at newsstands. I didn't know the lower extremity was cultivated taste in Japan. The American docs at the conference were blown away. We assumed it was porn! Imagine igniting amour with a tiny, stinky tootsie! The guys tried to be sleuths—to delicately inquire local physicians over dinner out of respect—but no one came away the wiser."

Waiting, being present, and encouraging an individual to expand on her story temporarily relieved heartache.

When I greeted her at our next session, Dr. Dunn mischievously smiled and stuck the book she was reading into her purse. Color had returned to her face. Lustrous pageboy locks brushed her cobalt Moroccan shawl. I noticed she walked with a perky stride. What a striking contrast from Monday's appointment. My curiosity was piqued.

I decided not to get rid of everything after all. We fashioned a hearty selection of the best drawings and photos and arranged them in brown packing paper. Ollie inscribed the date and a clever note on top. 'Caution: Twentieth-century sprites abided in this bungalow. Evidence within.' Then she took my pinkie, licked it succulently, and placed it on the center of the twine before tying a couple of bundles together. We stowed the goods back behind the rafters. Friendly ghosts roiled our juices just as that storm hit! I love hail.

Stumbling Upon Phantoms and Ghosts

To some extent, discovering a secret in one's family of origin or among those closest to us can be experienced as happening upon an unwanted ghost. You wish you had never seen it. The encounter lingers. The phantom's presence bubbles into consciousness at the most inopportune moments. It doesn't let go. You try to escape.

How could Dr. Dunn or I have predicted that over a weekend of clearing out her family's vacation home she would lose her emotional footing upon uncovering a trove of drawings and photographs hidden behind a false wall and in closets and the attic? Something provoked fragility and extreme backlash in this sturdy, resilient woman. I wondered whether psychotherapy always catalyzed a process of revealing one's own ghosts, such as Dr. Dunn's confession that she stowed away a private collection of her own in her garage for years, or her fascination with the titillating images she learned about on her business trip to Japan. Is the resurfaced residue worth acknowledging and processing, as opposed to simply trying to suppress it?

While it is impossible to know when a psychological ghost may emerge in our life, it's unlikely we will avoid encountering some. When that encounter inevitably happens, we can become so haunted that we are thrown off our stride and don't know where to turn next.

Secrets and ghosts are kindred spirits. I explain to patients that they walk together, but ghosts are felt in and by our body, often subliminally. So it's often hard to put our finger on what is going on inside or to name the experience in the moment. Both impact the body, but ghostly presences and intrapsychic phantoms are embodied phenomena: repercussions wielded by the full spectrum of our physical sensory-motor perceptions, experiences, and memories. "I got the willies," "felt nauseous," "itchy, tight skin," "scummy and slimy all over," "shivery, like I was five-year-old watching a horror movie," "had to watch my step more than once," and "couldn't catch my breath" are some of the phrases I have heard patients use to describe the uncanny experience of encountering a spectral presence.

Both secrets and ghosts take time to unpack because they come to life on the conscious-unconscious continuum. They can cause anxiety or anger to simmer—these are precisely the signals that prompt us to seek refuge by staying tight-lipped or displacing our feelings onto something or someone else. A displaced backlash of retribution can strike a serious and unwanted blow in a relationship, so we surreptitiously and unwittingly enact what is stirred up with those closest to us. We may try to move on temporarily, but the ghost stays lodged within until the secrets it holds emerge—as occurred with Dr. Dunn—or until further understood and worked through by the individual.

Psychodynamic psychotherapy is one opportunity that allows time and space to synthesize the nearly universal kind of short-lived and relatively benign traumatic encounters that Dr. Dunn experienced. Therapy can also help distinguish them from the less common but pernicious "multigenerational phantoms" and "transgenerational ghosts" she alluded to reading about in the contemporary psychoanalytic literature (Feldman, 2016; Grand, 2000, 2016; Harris, Kalb, & Klebanoff, 2016).

Sometimes ghosts awaken during psychotherapy, a side effect of the healing process that requires considerable effort and "tincture of time" to ameliorate.

While I believe that finding a good match in psychotherapy is invaluable in working through these situations, the treatment of transgenerational hauntings and multigenerational phantoms has notable differences from the work Dr. Dunn and I were doing at this juncture. Distinguishing features arise with other examples later in this chapter. Scenario work affords another look at how we understand and process the impact of ghosts and phantoms we may uncover in our lives. It gives us additional perspective on an essential question posed throughout the book: How does psychotherapy help alleviate psychic pain? Further, we might ask, what is the evidence that it does what it alleges to do?

What Ours Ghosts Teach Us about Life

It's striking how often scary ghosts outnumber friendly ones in fiction, the horror movie genre, and most cultures. Psychoanalytic theory posits that this occurs because in earliest childhood, we are helpless creatures in need of protection. To feel secure, we rely upon our caretakers to help us through all the sounds and sights that can and do go bump in the night. It's another testament to Dr. Dunn's secure early family environment, capacity for resilience, and previous analytic work that she can quickly begin to right the dysregulating experience of finding her family's "pornography," then put it into the perspective of our shared humanity, vulnerability, and idiosyncratic quirkiness.

A revision of our internal pictures of family members or aspects of our personal history can happen quickly. It is a challenge to integrate the new stock of stories into those we have told ourselves for decades about ourselves and those we love. When disclosed verbally—excavating physical evidence of the long withheld, forgotten, or buried—a secret can tarnish reputations and overturn idealizations. A serious rewrite of how we see and understand our relationships is indicated. Not infrequently, significant psychological turmoil erupts, and internal balance is temporarily overturned.

The opportunity to speak frankly and safely about what Dr. Dunn found shocking and shameful about family members, and the intertwined memories awakened from her career, quickly turned into a positive opportunity for playfulness and an erotic interlude. Between just two psychotherapy appointments—over about 72 hours—she snared the indelible, creepy apparitions. They emerged, almost magically transmogrified as benevolent helpers, in her relationship with her spouse Ollie. While quick turnarounds like this are rare in psychotherapy, the discovery of a family ghost prompts many to take a plunge into their psyche and a familial history that had been shrouded.

Just as Dr. Dunn had to reckon with this after a long career as keeper of her patients' confidences—part-time doctor at a women's prison, lifelong learner, traveler, and intimate partner to Ollie—every human being has unspoken needs and desire. These can be perplexing and overwhelming, but often quite pleasurable and exciting, to discover. It's no secret for any adult in the twenty-first century that it's not just those housed behind bars who "do weird stuff to get off." She was so shocked to find "the porn" in several corners of her life that her unconscious idealization of family members came to the surface. Her associations with what she stowed for years in her garage led her to grapple with just how common it is to denigrate and ward off from consciousness aspects of one's own life that simultaneously fascinate and give pleasure—in this case, the erotic objects of others.

Ego strength, including resolve and humor, is what allowed this patient to step back and own disavowed parts of herself while acknowledging foibles and disappointment of certain family members. The purpose of the therapy at this moment was to help her sort through something we all inherently know about others but rarely think about until a situation brings us up short. There are always chambers in the human heart, felt most acutely for those we love or place on a pedestal, that we will never fully know or comprehend. This can make us feel childlike, belittled, frustrated, or duped when we discover their secret.

Another Perspective on the Goal of Psychotherapy

One of the most apt and poetic descriptions of the entire psychotherapy process is found in the classic writings of analyst Hans Loewald. His thoughts are often summarized by teachers of psychotherapy as a process of "turning our ghosts into ancestors." The excruciating work of becoming aware of our ghosts facilitates healthier choices to claim and nurture our autonomous selves. Each of us must then struggle to decide what to hold on to and what to toss, which change to resist and which to embrace.

While both patient and therapist are gratified when such a metamorphosis happens (and particularly when it is sustained over time), experience dictates that fast relief is more the exception than the rule, particularly when withheld secrets, often encased in traumatic memories, must be metabolized. Only then can the heavy weights be shed. The past worth preserving is kept and, to some extent, reimagined and reinvested. We are then freed to derive strength and stability from our ancestors. Another patient of mine grasped this process with a lovely visual metaphor: "It's like a dense fog lifts. I see my path more clearly now."

Psychodynamic psychotherapists and psychoanalysts have many ways of formulating how this internal process of assimilation happens: it depends on our preferred theories or what makes clinical sense at the time. But the power of the therapeutic relationship can never be undersold. The therapist accompanies the patient through the ebbs and tides as she delves deeper into the personal inheritance of her newly discovered ghosts. As we hear in Dr. Dunn's associations, recognizing the humanity of others began to catalyze a fuller acceptance and transformation of herself. For her emotional equilibrium to be restored and her self-agency to flourish, she began to claim a veritable onslaught of thoughts and experiences she initially externalized.

At this juncture, the process has just begun. For its generative force to continue, Dr. Dunn would need to mourn old idealizations requiring ongoing wresting with her tangled feelings and conflicts. The discontinuity in self-experience generates a force field that comes alive in the therapeutic relationship. In that protected space, new information can be integrated with what one already knows and accepts about oneself. As Loewald goes on to explain in one of his classic papers, the therapist is active partner to the patient, who must ultimately take personal responsibility for reconning

with all that has been disavowed. Indeed, those inner hauntings often take on a life of their own in fantasy regardless of the external circumstances or traumas that gave rise to them:

> Those who know ghosts tell us that they long to be released from their ghost life and led to rest as ancestors. As ancestors they live forth in the present generation, while as ghosts they are compelled to haunt the present generation with their shadow life. . . In the daylight of analysis the ghosts of the unconscious are laid and led to rest as ancestors whose power is taken over and transformed into the newer intensity of present life. . . the unconscious needs present day external reality. . . and psychic reality. . . lest it be condemned to live the shadow life of ghosts or to destroy life.
>
> (1960, pp. 28–29)

Psychotherapy helps by securing the space for us to gather the split-off parts of ourselves and look at them in the light of day. Those shadows may not be as shameful, noxious, or heinous as we believe them to be in fantasy because they are part of the fabric of human nature. Discovering one's ghosts is a lifelong project, however. Psychotherapy neither immunizes against adult trauma or loss nor begets flawless human beings.

Every time we discover a new ghost over the course of life, we have an opportunity to grow into a truer version of ourselves. In a sense, this is what is meant by the old psychoanalytic aphorism that therapy helps by "making the unconscious conscious." Notice again that in Dr. Dunn's case, the discovery of erotic family pictures led her to associations and stories in the therapy that were not conscious at the beginning of the session but that she no longer warded off—laying to rest secrets and ghosts of her own that she had harbored for years and finding in the recollection newfound strands of strength, empathy, and perspective for herself and her loved ones.

We are tasked with rediscovering our internal "good objects" and leaning upon them to remain active agents in our adult development. This doesn't mean that one needs a therapist in perpetuity to help dispense with ghosts. The tools gathered in the process are portable, durable, and reusable. Should one encounter stumbling blocks, it's wise to return for another "chapter" of psychotherapy or analysis. When severe traumatic experience or multigenerational trauma is part of one's legacy, revisiting becomes essential.

Encountering Multigenerational Phantoms

What Dr. Dunn refers to as multigenerational phantoms and intergenerational ghosts is the specific clinical situation we turn to next. These issues are

receiving long-overdue attention in contemporary psychoanalysis because studies of genocide, racism, refugee crises, and war in all corners of our world have uncovered how traumatized groups pass on unconscious and therefore unmetabolized psychological trauma to the next generations. These studies are interdisciplinary in nature. Researchers in sociology, anthropology, history, biography, genetics, epigenetics, medicine, and psychoanalysis are coming together as never before to uncover the toxic effects on individual patients, groups, and nations who have undergone extraordinary degrees of violence, dislocation, forced immigration, and war (Apprey, 1998, 1999, 2014a, b; Leuzinger-Bohleber, 2021; Volkan, 1984, 1999, 2007, 2017). The losses incurred are mind-boggling, inevitably stirring ghostly presences and casting indelible shadows on body and psyche that can and often do take the form of physical and psychiatric illness.

When Dr. Maurice Apprey—professor at the University of Virginia School of Medicine, a psychoanalyst and expert on transgenerational hauntings—was interviewed about his research, he observed:

> I have come to see through clinical work and also in the communal memory of traumatized groups how humans carry errands to reduce themselves to ashes or derivatives thereof at the behest of their ancestral transgressors . . . . I have observed echoes of the phenomena in anorexia nervosa, gender identity disorder, some criminal psychopathic conditions, and the larger societal arena . . . groups that have undergone massive trauma such as African Americans, Holocaust survivors and so on.
> (Apprey, interview by Basseches, 1988, p. 15)

Because layers of trauma that hark back to prior generations are implicated in this wide swath of psychological disturbance, mental health professionals see firsthand how they gobble up enormous quantities of psychological energy. While concepts such as multigenerational hauntings, transgenerational transmission of trauma, psychic enclaves, psychic crypts, the illness of mourning, and unconscious errands have much to teach us about secrets and the devastating consequences they can sometimes cause in lives, they are qualitatively different from the story of Dr. Dunn. The sheer magnitude and repetition of the multigenerational and intergeneration trauma wreaks significant havoc on both the psyche and the soma. By way of contrast, the secret that Dr. Dunn uncovered was relatively innocuous and worked through quickly.

The slow, painful work of understanding and releasing concealed knowledge and devastating loss of hitherto "unspeakable secrets" (Torok, 1968; Abraham & Torok, 1972/1994; Raskin, 1992, 2008) can be one of the life-saving outcomes of psychodynamic psychotherapy or psychoanalysis too. At the group and societal level, application of psychodynamic concepts is being used to mediate ethnonational conflicts and to reconcile—and sometimes help redress and alleviate decades of grievance and injustice.

Although beyond the scope of this book, this ongoing research and its application to geopolitical hostilities are important to mention not only because of the good they attempt to accomplish for our fellow human beings worldwide but because they demonstrate a further proof of concept. There are aspects of personal history, trauma, bereavement, and stigma an individual might consider too shameful and unbearable to be shared with anyone. While secrets can have horrific impact on individuals or a group, what is masked and hidden becomes imperative in certain situations for psychic survival. A central question emerges in each unique situation: What are the psychological and somatic costs of well-kept but ultimately destructive secrets?

Diving Deeper: The Contributions of Nicolas Abraham and Maria Torok

The psychological underpinning of what is subsumed under the rubric of psychic phantoms, ghosts, demons, vampires, and dybbuks is emerging with renewed interest after a relatively quiescent period of clinical dismissal and disinterest. The Parisian analysts Nicolas Abraham and Maria Torok are two pioneers who published several groundbreaking papers and books on "the illness of mourning" in the 1960s and 1970s that first brought the phenomena of intrapsychic crypts to light. Their ideas derived from prior grounding in philosophy, world literature, and, most importantly, their ongoing investigation from clinical practice with survivors of severe trauma.

Abraham and Torok found that for many individuals, traumatic experiences could be neither assimilated nor mourned (Abraham & Torok, 1972, 1975). This starkly contrasted with some of Freud's most important observations and recommendations on assisting the grieving process. The two latter analysts strove to explain the conditions under which mourning became interminable.

The Holocaust, physical dislocation, and experiences of surviving innumerable deaths after both world wars provided an ample cohort of European patients whose psychological breakdown occurred because they did not move through the expectable passageways of loss. Remains of loved ones were often never found, and survivors were also deprived of their homeland by forced relocation. Psychologically speaking, the loved one could never be put to rest by the usual rites of funerals and periodic visitation; instead, they remained secretly entombed within individual and family psyches. For these survivors, the dead remained eternally, and uncannily, alive.

Unexplained physical illness, states of unreachable apathy, ennui, sorrow, and futility, eating disorders and starvation states, and chronic suicidal and murderous impulses were some of the intractable psychiatric conditions that Abraham and Torok found exemplify the illness of mourning. After the trauma, afflicted individuals were too ashamed and defeated to speak about their horrifying experiences openly. They sought, somewhat successfully, to house their memories unconsciously in what they conceptualized as a "psychological vault or crypt" (Rand, 1994a, b; Torok, 1968). The words are apt. The effects are rarely stored as discrete memories but are hidden in the deeper layers of the unconscious, where they remain isolated, denied, disavowed, dissociated from reality and, crucially, wordless. Amassed within the body unrelieved by the grieving process, the "exquisite corpse" is sensed as an empty space, vague sensation, or tense unsettling (Abraham & Torok, 1973, 1975; Rand, 1994a, b; Torok, 1968).

Sometimes what was lost—perhaps a deceased loved one or one's homeland—is experienced as a foreign body lodged within an "enclave" that inhibits growth and individuation (Abraham & Torok, 1994). This prevents the individual from moving on in life while simultaneously serving a protective psychological function by silencing the original catastrophe of devastating loss. The crypt preserves:

> Intact an unspeakable secret . . . (an) ineffable sense of unarticulated suffering. . .
>
> The ability to verbalize a secret signifies rather that the subject has surmounted an obstacle to being and can now reengage in the (still challenging) process of going-on-being. Such verbalizing also prevents a silenced drama from being transmitted transgenerationally to subjects who have had no direct experience of it . . . (and) who therefore cannot engage actively with it—either to resist or assimilate it—without some mediating agency or form of analytic investigation.
>
> (Raskin, 2008, pp. 21, 20)

The formulation and clinical recommendations of Abraham and Torok have been of inestimable value to many clinicians working with individuals and groups who experienced catastrophic trauma. Applying their ideas helps us further understand secrets' multifarious ramifications on individuals who have undergone more travail than Dr. Dunn, yet are not as psychologically annihilated as survivors of cataclysmic events, when truth and personal history cannot be spoken.

We now turn to a case in point: the psychotherapy of Margaretta, a patient I treated over two decades ago, who vivified Nicolas Abrahams's aphorism, "What haunts are not the dead, but the gaps left within us by the secrets of others" (Abraham, 1975, p. 171). The phrase he coined helps explain how a missing link sensed in a treatment process may emanate from a source other than the designated patient—and is intuited by embodied experience and countertransference resonance by the therapist.

Discovering Psychic Crypts in the Consulting Room

Margaretta, age fifty-eight, entered psychotherapy several years after her husband had been killed in an accident.[2] The couple had no children. She received significant gratification from working in the business that she and her husband had established together, although she acknowledged that her confidence and sense of self had a tendency to flag, despite the outward accomplishment. At the time of her husband's death, the business had been on a firm foundation, and Margaretta was ready to change direction in her life. She had a long-term but seemingly unreachable goal to start a not-for-profit agency to assist migrants and victims of human trafficking in her hometown in the Midwest.

When she began psychotherapy, Margaretta was grieving. Her bereavement was so intense that she could barely speak, let alone share any personal history. Listless, unable to sleep, and preoccupied with guilt, she agreed to my suggestion to begin medication immediately. Her initial symptoms quickly improved, and she decided to continue twice-weekly psychotherapy to explore what might have blocked her sense of agency throughout her life.

Margaretta had few ideas about what was holding her back: her husband had always supported her goals. She told me she held out the possibility of dating someday but felt this would be disloyal to her deceased spouse.

As Margaretta began to open up a bit more, I learned that her adoring and admired father was often away on business trips in her childhood and adolescence. The oldest of four children, she recalled close ties with each parent until she began middle school. Margaretta's mother had a sudden personality change: she complained of constant pain, became addicted to painkillers, experienced rapid emotional shifts, and continually berated her children. Overcome with tears as she confided the bullying, Margaretta said she believed her mother hated her and accused her of "being ugly, evil, stupid, and the cause of all my problems."

To complicate matters further, Margaretta's grandparents died before she entered her teens; they had been important ancillary attachment figures who provided a safe haven for the siblings on weekends. According to Margaretta, her parents never discussed the losses with the children. I began to suspect that her husband's death had excavated unprocessed grief about the grandparents and rage at mother that could not be verbalized at the time. I speculated that Margaretta had incorporated her mother's disparaging images that interfered with her creative living and perpetuated an illness of mourning. Moreover, I wondered whether one or more secrets led to her mother's decompensation that were unwittingly transmitted to the patient who

> Reenacts dramas of shame, fear, or disgrace that evoke and concretize these silent traumas. . . (and) the unstated obligation to keep the secret invisible and unreachable. . . as a necessary means of maintaining the parent's and the family's integrity.
>
> (Raskin, 2008, p. 106)

Keeping in mind the clinical insights of Abraham and Torok, I inferred that the tenacity of Margaretta's symptoms, which included unrelenting bereavement and somatic complaints, might be understood as aspects of her parents and grandparents that were entombed in her psyche. Perhaps these intrapsychic crypts reflected intergenerational trauma that foreclosed mourning? Had she incorporated her mother to such an extent as to think of herself in the same way her mother had? A phantom was concealed and must be psychologically exorcised in the therapy for her to move on. What could Margaretta be withholding from the past that needed to be recognized and further processed?[3]

I pointed out some of the good things her mother had also given to her in her youth. No one was all good or bad, and I proposed that Margaretta and her mother had a similar struggle: they both wanted to be better at giving and receiving love than they had allowed themselves to be. I asked whether there were any inklings that mother had experienced abuse, trauma, or catastrophic upheaval such as war or forced migration. I knew I was making a stab in the dark, but I had confidence that Margaretta would let me know if I was off the beam.

After these simple, and to some obvious, conjectures to help engage and clarify, I was caught off guard. Margaretta let out a ghostly and unexpected howl. It appeared to have unlocked a crypt. She said,

> I have kept this memory to myself for years. I didn't think anyone would believe it. I was in the hospital room when my mother died. A mysterious warmth came over me and I knew she really loved me at that moment. I also immediately recognized that she found me pretty and competent. *It was my secret.* I didn't want to tell you.

The first psychic crypt that Margaretta unlocked was the unspoken love she and her mother had for each other. It was quite moving to witness Margaretta excavating the entombed experience of love that had laid silently beneath the manifest hatred she consciously and effortlessly spoke about in the treatment. My lucky guess might have provided the unconscious permission she needed in her psychic reality to divulge what she considered to be

> A crazy wish for some kind of benevolent afterlife . . . although I do know it to be true—that is, what my mother conveyed during my solitary vigil. She did love me and admired what I did in my life.

Something important still seemed to be left unsaid. I was curious about the emphasis placed on physical attractiveness in this family, in part because of my experience working with eating disorder patients. Well into treatment, I often found that earlier generations of women in the family of origin were preoccupied with shape, weight, eating, beauty standards, activity levels, and the like for unknown reasons. Anorexia, bulimia, and binge eating did not begin with the Baby Boomer generation, nor are they only sustained by social media, cultural injunctions, and biological diatheses (Lapid, Chen, Rummins, McAlpine, et al., 2013; Wooldridge, 2018; Zerbe, 1993/1995, 2001, 2007, 2008, 2016; Zerbe, Becker, & Yager, 2002; Zerbe & Satir, 2016).

Had another insidious message been passed on to Margaretta that stymied her sense of self-worth? What secret or mystery might be contained within that, once released, could spark additional emotional expression and, eventually, greater psychological freedom? As Abraham and Torok described, some children of Holocaust survivors developed severe anorexia. The parent who was starved in the camps and unable to expose the shame, trauma, and guilt about what happened to them found unconscious ways to transmit it to their child, who lived it out. So one formulation that I took into consideration in the treatment of Margaretta was that her self-esteem pathology—although she did not have an eating disorder—was a mask for her mother's suffering. Were there traumas that her mother had weathered? Had a body image problem, eating disturbance, or other psychiatric issue passed into, through, and become transposed in my patient from something her mother had concretely suffered? It's a riveting but important gem of an insight that each of us might consider as we reflect on our ongoing mental well-being and some ghosts we may harbor:

> Symptoms do not spring from the individual's own life experiences but from someone else's psychic conflicts, traumas, or secrets . . . the dead do not return, but their lives' unfinished business is unconsciously handed down to descendants. . . laying the dead to rest and cultivating our ancestors implies uncovering their shameful secrets, understanding their nameless and undisclosed suffering.
>
> (Rand, 1994b, pp. 166–167)

The second psychic crypt opened only after I pressed for more information about Margaretta's understanding of her mother's penchant for verbal abuse that focused on physical appearance. Gradually, she revealed a hidden discovery. After her parents' deaths in the late 1970s, she found her mother's diary and became interested in conducting genealogy research. She unearthed documentation of a multigenerational eating disorder and preoccupation with beauty standards in several female relatives. A great aunt in the 1920s had been a film star, noted for her physical beauty and charm. One family myth was, "Everyone has a legacy. Live up to this one."[4]

This previously undisclosed throughline helped us make sense of the verbal castigation Margaretta endured in adolescence. Her mother had transmitted a phantom of her own: the experience of feeling unattractive and not measuring up to the standards of her aunt. The comparison filled pages of her mother's musings in journals and letters. The dangerous secret of a multigenerational eating disorder or addiction within a family layered over conflict, dysfunction, and alienation precludes trust and open dialogue, as it had in this sad situation (Imber-Black, 1998; Krestan & Bepko, 1993; Roberto, 1993; Zerbe, 1993/1995, 2001, 2008, 2016).

Margaretta and I surmised that her mother's feelings about this burden ran deep. Her mother's somatic illness, drug abuse, and harangues were faulty attempts to cure herself. The secrets had been transmitted to Margaretta, who carried them for all these years in the form of a feeling that she should not "use her mouth" to speak for herself; her mother's trauma was concealed but passed on to her. Now we could begin to put the story into words in the therapy. This catalyzed a mourning process, a first step in removing obstacles for healing, personal growth, and individuation.

Through the Lens of Contemporary Psychotherapy Research: Transgenerational Trauma and Its Treatment

Marianne Leuzinger-Bohleber is a training and supervising analyst in the German Psychoanalytical Association and former director of the Sigmund Freud Institute in Frankfort, Germany. Her interdisciplinary, international research collaborative brings together neuroscientists, cognitive scientists, practicing therapists and analysts, and developmental researchers. It entails clinical and extraclinical research arms to help achieve a better understanding of how to treat patients with an array of psychiatric disorders and, ultimately, how to prevent them.

In Germany, where three-times-weekly intensive psychotherapy and psychoanalysis are supported by generous government insurance, there is ongoing necessity to demonstrate its value and cost effectiveness to the population. Leuzinger-Bohleber's "plurality of methods" includes randomized controlled trials and the single-case-study method (Leuzinger-Bohleber, 2008, 2015a). The goal is to improve the mental health system as a whole and delineate the best treatment method for the individual. This research is ongoing but has already demonstrated the efficacy of psychodynamic treatment in patients with chronic depression, psychogenic infertility, post-polio syndrome and other somatic disorders, and trauma.

In one notable case study, Leuzinger-Bohleber describes a woman in her research cohort who had intractable depression (Leuzinger-Bohleber, 2015a). The patient she calls Ms. B. had undergone many attempts at pharmacotherapy and individual psychotherapy. Her extreme psychosomatic symptoms led her to enter Leuzinger-Bohlelber's study and to begin thrice-weekly psychoanalysis as a last resort.

In the psychoanalytic treatment, Ms. B. gradually came to appreciate that her abusive mother had lost both of her own parents during the First World War and sorted through the subterranean ways it pummeled her mother's childhood and adolescence. Ms. B's father was a Nazi soldier. He went missing in her early years, assumed to be killed in combat or taken prisoner on the Eastern Front, only to reemerge in the early 1950s.[5] The patient had no sense of stable identity; she fused with her paternal grandmother and mother, whom she tried to appease by false compliance. Although Ms. B. had minimal contact with her father until she was in late midlife, she idealized him. In the context of repeated rape by an uncle and sexual promiscuity in young adulthood, a bevy of psychosomatic symptoms arose, including migraine headaches, sleep issues, and eating disorders. As the patient put it to her analyst, "I have no sense of who I really am" (2015a, pp. 76–77).

Within the treatment, this patient had to confront the disavowed "rage, anger, and hate" that she projected repeatedly onto her analyst. Leuzinger-Bohleber believes that the analyst's ability to sustain formidable and repeated verbal attacks was paramount in helping Ms. B. gain a sense of perspective and find a new and robust sense of self-agency. This patient's resilience enabled her to make use of the psychoanalytic treatment, to eventually establish a satisfying marriage, and to free herself from the physical pain of her embodied memories. First, she had to reclaim her mother's traumatic past that had been long buried. This meant discussing family secrets and her mother's sequestered but conscious personal history.

During analysis, the patient had many painful conversations with her mother that confirmed the multiple traumas and rapes that both her maternal grandmother and mother sustained during World War I. These recounted narratives enabled Ms. B. to "sever the 'depressive umbilical cord'" (p. 78) between herself and her mother; she was starting to be able to differentiate her needs and feelings from theirs. The patient slowly recognized that she was unconsciously replaying her mother's past in her own life and that it was getting in the way of living her own. Moreover, the embodied memories that had caused her physical pain and somatic illnesses could now be understood as "deposited" into her from her caretakers who transmitted their trauma and unresolved losses into her. Psychological and physical well-being improved gradually over the years she was in treatment and was sustained at follow-up.

Leuzinger-Bohleber emphasizes in her publications that while more

> Clinical and extra-clinical research is needed . . . we have learned from our prevention studies that we need to focus on the transgenerational dimensions of aggression, antisocial, and depressive behavior of children at risk . . . real prevention will only be effective if we succeed in also reaching the traumatized parents.
>
> (p. 79)

Learning about the transmission of trauma from one generation to the next in their family of origin helped other subjects in the DPV and LAC studies disrupt a vicious cycle. These beneficiaries of psychodynamic treatment parented their children differently from the way they were parented. They used their newfound knowledge and reflective capabilities to help themselves appreciate and withstand the developmental requirements posed by the stresses and strains of raising their children.

The unexpected findings of studies over the last decades show that "the connection between trauma and depression is much more dramatic than the classical psychoanalytical literature had postulated" (p. 51). But that connection can be modified for beneficent effects when historical reality that "remains preserved in these narrations and must be understood in order to introduce sustainable processes of psychic transformation" (p. 91) is expressed during trusting, in-depth therapy. The DPV and LAC research groups speculate that epigenetic patterns can ultimately be modified to diminish an array of tenacious and heretofore refractory psychological symptoms. This remains one of the central goals of psychodynamic treatment.

Concluding Observations from a Spy's Daughter: Sara Taber's *Born under an Assumed Name*

Clinical examples like Leuzinger-Bohleber's Ms. B may seem distant from contemporary reality. Even experienced clinicians who work with transgenerational trauma born from the long-term consequences of American slavery, the Holocaust, Argentina's Dirty War, the Armenian genocide, and South Africa's apartheid find the work psychologically grueling to body and mind because the ghosts, phantoms, and shadows reverberate (Apprey,

1999, 2006, 2014b; Volkan, 2013). They have learned that tensions in large groups can be ameliorated to some extent, but because they are complex and multigenerational, they are rarely extinguished. The role of witness to pernicious trauma is frequently experienced as excruciating. The noxious effects and emotional residuals are hard to perceive or fully fathom. As much as the therapist or facilitator of a sociopolitical reconciliation team consciously wants to help, a protective counterforce emerges to shove the stories of maltreatment and horror out of mind. Mind-body dissociation and somatic reactivity in the witness or therapist may be one thorny consequence.[6]

Recently, psychoanalysis has begun to be more mindful about how clinicians must address our own wellness and vulnerability to sustain ourselves over time—this likely applies to other secret keeping professions too (Harris & Sinsheimer, 2008; Maroda, 2022; Zerbe, 2022b). Being present for persons exposed to transgenerational trauma and multigenerational hauntings sometimes means taking advantage of a normative defense that psychoanalyst Richard Druss (1995, 2000) called "healthy denial." Uncovering and casting light on shadows and putting intrapsychic ghosts to rest comes at a price that may go unseen by therapist and patient alike. As discussed, individuals can appear to put thoughts and feelings about secrets on the backburner, but they have a way of searing their way into our unconscious, disrupting the capacity to think clearly and to remain grounded and resilient.

Transgenerational transmission of trauma seen in the consulting room and experienced by individuals and family members is not always the result of international catastrophe and upheaval or caused by attachment insecurity or childhood maltreatment. In a riveting memoir, social worker and author Sara Mansfield Taber describes the legacy she endured growing up as a spy's daughter. She looks backward from the present to her childhood and adolescence in *Born under an Assumed Name: The Memoir of a Cold War Spy's Daughter* (2012) to understand her current life.

Taber is resolutely respectful of and grateful for the rich opportunities she had in her youth: she colorfully details growing up in different countries where she imbibed diverse, fascinating cultural experiences that most of us would envy. Her dual careers in mental health services and writing are no doubt shaped by what she gleaned during her formative years that later fed her ability to nurture what she calls a "penchant for complex and oblique truths, and a built-in, sensitive secret detector" (p. 248). The reader is left to ponder the complicated and difficult truth that Taber, until her twenties, had no conscious awareness of—that her father was living a double life as an American spy who worked for the CIA.

In the memoir, Taber describes a severe psychotic episode that took her by storm in late adolescence while going to school in Japan. She experienced unremitting high fever and severe headache. Her illness persisted, and its etiology remained mysterious despite extensive medical workup and superior medical care at an American military hospital in Japan. After recovery, she was embarrassed to tell others about what happened, and she wondered what effect the knowledge would eventually have on her future spouse and children. Taber's psychiatrist intervened by offering her seemingly perfunctory but wise advice: "try honesty" and to "face her fears" (p. 321). Had he been intuiting all along that his patient was holding back essential self-knowledge and vital personal history that was the source of her creative inhibition, self-reproach, and dysphoria?

Psychosis thrust Taber into an identity crisis. She became aware in group therapy sessions in the hospital that the sense of self she concocted for herself was false. Although she never directly defines her plight as one of transgenerational trauma per se (perhaps unaware of the terminology), gaps in her awareness, disorientation, secrecy, need to perpetually stay on the move as an adult, and capacity to endure unconscious, embodied memories are descriptive features illustrated throughout the text of "Living under a Shadow of Ghosts" (Durban, 2016, pp. 81–83) of a prior generation or existent family member (i.e., transgenerational trauma). Taber's psychiatrist eventually concluded that her psychosis was caused by an allergy to over-the-counter ephedrine. While psychosis caused by an illicit substance is common in psychiatry, Taber reportedly ingested something that is usually innocuous; in fact, its parent compound—epinephrine—is ubiquitous in the body and vital for survival. One is left to speculate whether the drug itself or the way it was manufactured was the sole cause of her delirium or if the need for psychiatric care was considerably more complicated.

Given the consequences to her and her family members, the price of her father's career is always a question. As a child, Taber idealized her father, who told his children that he worked for a US government agency. He encouraged her and her younger brother to pursue their abilities, played with them, and paid attention to their interests. Yet something lurked in the shadows; there were parts of her own life and her father's that she could never grasp. To achieve wellness, she concludes at the end of her memoir that she eventually had

> To face the miasma of our secrets, stoicism, and false identities. And beyond the obvious secrets and fake identities we'd long harbored deeper ones with which we had to come to grips: the secrets of our human needs and vulnerability.
>
> (p. 321)

She believes that her father's severe depression, which worsened after retirement, and her parents' marriage difficulties, which led to eventual divorce, were caused by years of mutual dissembling because "hiding himself had become a habit he couldn't break" (p. 246).

Taber's younger brother, on the other hand, was not surprised by their father's eventual revelations. And her mother was aware of her husband's profession and helped him remain undercover wherever they lived. Once again, a secret life had been "hidden, but in plain view," although Taber denies having any conscious inkling of it. Like so many of my patients who must confront a long-buried family secret and then blurt out in therapy, "suddenly, everything came together and made sense to me," Taber perceives the consequences of what was never spoken and what she could not allow herself to know when she writes these passages:

> I didn't know how dangerous emotions were in my parents' world. I didn't know the pressures on them, how my father's job was—surreptitiously, clandestinely—destroying parts of them. How my mother had to control her emotions all the time. How my father was going underground with his, and the submerging would turn into an undertow.
>
> (p. 240)

> Beware of secrets . . . The romance of secrecy walks hand in hand with the headlongness of aggression . . . After my CIA childhood, I'd spend a lot of my life underground in one way or another. And truth would seem wavery, to dwell in the hidden.
>
> (p. 358)

Putting secrets and ghosts to rest by reconstructing a personal narrative activates psychological turbulence. Taber's account reminds us that the subjective experience of reality (what psychoanalysts call "psychic reality") is interwoven with what we recollect and reclaim in memory. Historical truth and our personal elaboration of that truth in fantasy are inextricably linked. Both are necessary to stake full claim to our common humanity, particularly our flaws and vulnerabilities. On this path, one has the opportunity to find a truer sense of oneself where creative potential and zest for life may blossom.

After their release from the brain's hazy divide along the conscious-unconscious continuum, secrets can be reworked to become less stultifying and shaming. As the examples in this chapter and Taber's memoir also illustrate, the gravitational force of a secret that pulls one down can be inverted by raising it to light and engaging with it in verbal dialogue or a creative act such as writing. These actions can ultimately transform the secret's power into the service of greater resilience and self-knowledge.

Conclusion

Secrets may take the form of an unwanted ghost or psychological phantom, which requires time for anyone to unpack. These ghosts are a challenge to integrate into the psyche because they occur on the conscious-unconscious continuum that manifests within the body. Some individuals in a family may be aware of the specific secret or hidden information, while others appear to be able to wall the knowledge off completely. This incongruence among family members is mysterious. When the ghost does emerge as an unassailable fact, the individual who confronts it has an opportunity to begin to make sense of their life in ways that were not available beforehand and that may simultaneously ameliorate some bamboozling, long-standing psychological difficulties and physical symptoms.

Homeostasis is temporarily overturned, whirlwind-like, when one begins to rewrite personal history unleashed by confronting ghosts and phantoms, a healing process that may be facilitated by a psychotherapist or confidant who serves as witness to the unfurrowing of the previously buried information. Inevitably, a process of mourning and wrestling with one's ambivalent feelings unfolds that ultimately catalyzes life forces. Layers of psychic pain are released when demons are laid to rest. But for many who suffer, the task remains so terrifying and difficult that unconscious defenses or conscious choices join forces to keep the apparitions entombed in an intrapsychic crypt. Clinical work and research studies document that manifestations of the intrapsychic crypt can block productivity and creativity, undergird unremitting depression as well as eating disorders and addictions, and even result in a plethora of undiagnosed somatic illnesses.

While they study individuals exposed to extraordinary levels of trauma through dislocation, forced immigration, war, and natural catastrophe, contemporary psychoanalysts are collaborating with interdisciplinary scholars from diverse fields to apply the concept of multigenerational phantoms and intergenerational ghosts to international conflict, political upheaval, and reconciliation efforts across the globe. The "unspeakable secrets" of the severely traumatized shed further light on the psychological and physical tolls experienced by those burdened with well-kept but ultimately destructive family secrets, often buried for generations.

Clinicians should remain on the lookout for transgenerational trauma in all patients, especially those with long-standing addiction and eating disorders, undiagnosed somatic problems, dissociation, depression, chronic PTSD, and other anxiety disorders that manifest themselves as embodied phenomena. These are the end result of the ghosts and phantoms that stay buried in the body's crypt. Integrating historical realities into one's life story appears to have a robust positive effect in the accumulated research studies and case reports to date and may play a significant preventive role in attenuating mental illness in the next generation.

Notes

1 For sage advice on how clinicians can stay grounded in extraordinary challenging situations that can temporarily dysregulate and stymie the capacity to think clearly about next steps in the treatment, see Peebles, M. J. (1983). Handling psychiatric urgency: Or, keeping one's diagnostic wits in a crisis. *Bulletin of the Menninger Clinic*, 47, 453–471. See also Peebles, M. J. (2022) for specific suggestions on approaching patients whose psychotherapy is not moving forward at the usual pace and who appear to be 'stuck'. Casting a wide net to include a swath of patients who do not quickly imporove, practical help is also afforded to readers who treat victims of transgenerational trauma where progress can move at a snail's pace, if at all, for long periods.

2 For a discussion of this case that emphasizes its impact on the therapist's somatic countertransference, see Zerbe, 2022.

3 I am grateful to Irwin C. Rosen, PhD, who pointed out that the concept of exorcism as a therapeutic metaphor was originally employed by Scottish psychoanalyst W.R.D. Fairbairn.

4 One cinematic example of transgenerational transmission of trauma is *The Good Shephard* (2006) in which the lead character (Matt Damon) takes on an unconscious errand after his father's suicide. Only at the end of the movie does Damon's character become aware of the cost of his career in the CIA and how the traumatic transmission of trauma impacted his wife, son, and himself.

5 This patient was one of the many depressed "children of war" whom Leuzinger-Bohleber encountered in the DPV (German Psychoanalytical Association Follow-Up) and LAC (Laboratory of Affect and Communication Study of Depression) studies she cites in her work (Leuzinger-Bohleber, 2008, 2015a, b, 2021; Leuzinger-Bohleber, Kallenbach, & Schoett, 2016; Leuzinger-Bohleber, Solms, & Arnold, 2020).

6 Traumatic transmission of trauma happens by many routes, including the professional life of one's parent. It's not only the progeny of spies who are afflicted. However, some additional illustrations can be found in Lucinda Franks (2007) *My father's secret war: A memoir*. New York: Hyperion (see Chapter 7); Mazower, M. (2017). *What you do not tell: A father's past and the journey home*. New York: Other Press; Richman, S. (2012). *A wolf in the attic: The legacy of a hidden child of the Holocaust*. New York: Routledge.

5 Somatic Countertransference

Hunter Allen, LCSW, had another splitting headache. He decided to seek consultation with me to discuss his patient Audra, whom he had been treating in twice-weekly psychotherapy for more than three years.

> While I can't predict when I will get one, they're getting more frequent. The pain only occurs when I see her—not with any other patient in my practice, or else I'd be worried something medical is going on. I suspect it's a somatic countertransference reaction. I can't put my finger on what it's about.

I leaned backward—likely grimacing, the giveaway that I was concerned about his health even though I hadn't said a word.

Hunter picked up on nonverbal signals.

> Yes, I checked in with my PCP. I was worried too. Everything is fine— only tension headaches. Maybe related to stress? I turn forty-two next year and the twins are starting grad school. Time is rolling along. My wife and I are thinking of adopting a puppy when our son finishes high school. Obvious way to plump the empty nest.

Glad his family was doing well, I asked him to tell me more about the case and why he returned to see me for consultation. We hadn't met for a supervision session since he finished his two-year postgraduate psychotherapy program prior to the COVID-19 pandemic.

"I love practice and teaching," he said,

> And I like Audra. She's thirty years old, married, a teacher. She's invested in treatment and works hard. But I find myself constantly questioning my interventions. Are my headaches telling me something important about what we're missing? It feels like I'm pulling out my teeth trying to figure this out.

DOI: 10.4324/9781003471578-6

It was a pleasure to see Hunter again and listen as he told me about the case. Over eight years, I had watched him grow from newly minted social worker to rock-solid clinician. His innate aptitude and confidence blossomed. He was open to learning from multiple sources. With hobbies like comedy performance, improv, and modern dance, he readily tuned in to his own and his patients' body cues. Sensory experience and physical reactivity were interests we both shared and discussed from time to time during his weekly supervision in the postgraduate training in psychodynamic psychotherapy.

I nodded in agreement. Hunter had made an important observation about a sensory phenomenon that occurred when he was with his patient Audra. I suggested he stay open to what his physical reactions might be telling him.

"Let the bodies in the room have time to speak for themselves and don't be in a rush to close down this conversation," I said.

"But how do I do that?" he interrupted. "It feels like I'm entering a torture chamber when I start the session because I don't know if I'll get one of those killer headaches. I know this sounds dramatic but it's the truth. I've started to wonder if I've come to the end of the line with what I can do. Do you think I should refer Audra to another therapist?" he asked.

"Let's try to stay curious for a little longer to wonder whether Audra might not be able to put into words what your body is tuning into," I replied. "Did you notice that you've used expressions like 'pulling teeth,' 'torture chamber,' 'killer' and 'dramatic'? I wonder if she's split off anger, aggression, or rage. Has she spoken about trauma or abuse in her history?"

"The more I try to suggest that she's angry or disappointed with me, the more she says I sound like a textbook. She denies abuse. She shuts me down."

"That hurts," I said. "She pushes you away and devalues you at the same time." I took a beat, quiet and still, to see where Hunter's thoughts might lead.

"I can take my share of negativity from patients but in her case it doesn't seem to fit," he elaborated. "I don't think she's angry. When you say let the body speak for itself, what do you mean? What do I do?"

There are many ways to investigate the body experience. Perhaps Audra too had headaches or other somatic responses. Hunter could ask Audra to take a "tour of her body" while they were together in session.

Hunter remembered Elvin Semrad's "tour of the body" technique, which I had taught in class.

I'll try. I remember feeling knots in my shoulders and back while I attempted to mentally circumnavigate my extremities and core during analysis. Such a weird response, but it did lead somewhere unexpected.

Remember the disgust I felt about my little sister? She's the one with cystic fibrosis who almost died when I was babysitting. I had to plunge a plastic tube down her throat over and over again to dislodge gobs of putrid gunk! She kept choking until my folks got home. It was thirty minutes of terror for both of us.

I did remember.

"With Audra I can work on being more attentive to breathing and tuning into physical sensations—hers and mine. It hasn't yielded anything yet, but it doesn't mean it won't."

I ended Hunter's consultation, curious about what ideas might percolate to the top of our conscious minds. Would Hunter and Audra be able to work through a stalemate that he sensed was causing his headaches? Would verbal processing be enough? How could Hunter gain additional access to the embodied phenomena he experienced? Perhaps a story was hiding in plain sight, one that Audra had not elaborated and that might lead to a place never before broached in the therapy.

The Consultation Sessions

Hunter and I met every other week to talk about his frustration with Audra's lack of progress. His headaches continued, but they bothered him less. Having a place to come and discuss the case had relieved his demoralization. Between meetings, we reviewed some contemporary papers on accessing body-mind reactivity, emphasizing the work of Norwegian psychoanalyst Jon Sletvold. Still, despite putting our heads together, nothing appeared to be moving in Audra's treatment.

One day, Hunter casually mentioned that he and his wife had started to take classes in ballroom dancing. "It livens me up and is great for our relationship," he said. "It brings back courtship memories." He reminded me about a continuous case seminar he had loved, called Bodies in the Session, that he took in the second year of his psychotherapy program. Students were encouraged to get in touch with their corporeal self. The instructor, a Los Angeles psychoanalyst and master at body-mind communication, had asked Hunter and his classmates to "pantomime the patient." Some students found the exercise annoying; others were amazed to watch how so much interpersonal information gets communicated without words. "Such a unique class," Hunter said. "And great fun for me, the improvisational entertainer!"

"Why not go with this train of thought now," I suggested.

I think this and your association to the dance lessons also mirrors some of our conversation about the case. Our reading about the body in psychotherapy may be tuning in to your recollections and lessons with your wife. You're a dancer! Take a couple of minutes after Audra finishes her session and pantomime the interaction that just occurred in your office. Think of it as another pathway—a nonverbal pathway—that might get you out of the muck. Use your imagination. See what happens. I'm here for you.

What Blocked Progress?

Sometimes, Hunter told me, after Audra's psychotherapy hour, he took a few private moments to "dance the session" as a mode of self-supervision. He pretended to be her, then transitioned to being himself in the role of therapist, and finally tried to create what he sensed might be happening jointly in the interpersonal space between them. He also took a few process notes about the content of what he and Audra said to each other. In our consultation process, he shared notes, imagining where her psychotherapy might be leading. As I remained a relatively quiet companion, he told the story, here relayed in full:

"It wasn't so much of a secret after all. How did I miss it? Audra simply didn't think it was important information to get into at this time of her life. We were working on anxiety and sadness after she received a promotion at the high school. The transition was a positive one but of course also meant letting go of teaching a couple of classes. We were discussing how she could balance the grueling hours of her husband's law practice and their desire to have a second baby.

When I took her initial history, Audra had skimmed over a rock-climbing accident she had in Yosemite when she was seventeen. Prior to the mishap, she had been a star athlete. Injuries to both legs required multiple surgeries over a couple of years—it upended her drive for extreme sport, which she sublimated into academic pursuits.

I don't know how I got there, but when I tried to dance her part after she left her session, I couldn't do it. One day I found myself getting irritated about this block. I wanted to pound my fists and swear. That's not like me. I took a step back to speculate what might not be getting enough airtime in the treatment. My body wasn't free to react in the dance. My paralysis in motion was telling me something.

I suddenly recalled the story about her accident, but we never delved into it. Duh. Until this moment she denied that she had leftover feelings about what had happened in her teens. I told her I had an idea I wanted to pose for each of us to think about and brought up the accident. I said that what happened was a trauma and the numerous medical procedures and loss of sports afterwards were repeated, albeit different types, of psychic wounds. I said I thought she dealt with the calamity by minimizing and shelving the residuals in her mind—shoulders back, chin up, stiff upper lip. While the defense helped get her though a very tough time, the consequences couldn't be shut off forever, and we needed to talk about the impact.

I realized I was taking a risk. I didn't harangue her, but I sensed I was onto something. I kept using the word 'trauma' with different modifiers in front: 'derailing,' 'unexpected,' 'painful.' Two words together opened flood gates. She's bringing it all in at last—a sense of untapped loss and loads of story fragments about her family and what happened after the fall.

And you know what? My headaches are better. They're not gone. I'm thinking about what my sister went through despite doing well after her lung transplant. That's where listening to Audra is taking me on a personal level. A sad slog through recollections. Part of my own history worming its way out like never before. Self-analysis. It never quits, does it?"

Tuning in to the Body's Reactivity

The clinician's body's reactivity is frequently the first harbinger of an unshared but crucial piece of the patient's narrative or an important detail of their history. It may not be fully explored or understood, but it can have significant meaning for the treatment. Hunter's patient Audra had not kept her adolescent accident a secret, but she had been able to defensively cordon off layers of its emotional impact. As we know by now, it is often this shadowy spiral of long suppressed feelings that gets in the way of the forward arc of treatment—toward living a full life.

At the moment of revelation, neither patient nor therapist can know whether this material has been dissociated, repressed, or deemed so unimportant that it need not be discussed. The precise defensive strategy—whether dissociation, repression, or something else—is nowhere near as important as the impact that disavowal has on the patient's body and one's own (Cramer, 2006; Wachtel, 2023; Zerbe, 1993/1995, 2008; Zerbe & Bradley, 2018; Zerbe & Satir, 2016). The patient's tangled webs of feelings and storyline may be split off from awareness but are essential to decode if relief is to be gained. An attuned therapist can use their own corporeal reactions as an additional point of access.

Hunter's intuitive and empathic capacities expanded during his postgraduate training and personal analysis, freeing him to recognize communications on the conscious-unconscious continuum that were going on between himself and Audra. After he made sure his recurring headaches were not a symptom of illness, the consultation process he and I underwent was a way to take stock of essential hurdles he encountered with Audra's treatment. He found additional guidance in appreciating Audra's experience of herself by using a technique recommended by Jon Sletvold.

Evidenced by his dancing after sessions, Hunter was able to attune to both bodies in the therapy room because he took embodied subjectivity seriously. He also did what Sletvold calls keeping "the you" of the other person in mind by embodying Audra in dance and then bringing both together intersubjectively: the "we" experience of embodied reflectivity (Sletvold, 2011, 2012, 2014, 2016; Sletvold & Brothers, 2021). It gave Hunter confidence to take his somatic countertransference (the headaches) seriously and to focus on an essential part of his patient's history (the accident) that was nebulous but substantially affecting her emotional life.

Hunter revealed in our meetings that he also discovered repressed feelings about his sister's illness that required further self-analysis, but he kept the therapeutic boundary with Audra and did not share this private information. By assuming different postures and points of view in the dance exercise, he engaged in what Sletvold calls a "two-body perspective" that shifts from mind to body, and then reverses gears from body to mind, to gain access to the subjectivities of each participant. Over several therapy sessions, the exercise led Hunter to formulate that Audra might be holding long-withheld feelings about the accident that were having residual, unspoken, and largely unacknowledged effects on her life. In contemporary parlance, this discovery enabled Hunter to bring to mind (mentalize) the helplessness and dread Audra did not want to reawaken that was nonetheless communicated between them, the first portent being Hunter's throbbing and persistent headaches.

Finding ways to tune in and take seriously one's somatic countertransference reactions is of resurging interest in the psychotherapy profession. Appreciating one's somatic (or embodied) countertransference can bring secrets or suppressed storylines to awareness because these narratives are also frequently housed within the body. The first procedure Hunter used to access what he sensed at the time was a somatic countertransference reaction was, in fact, a corporeal check-in procedure devised by Dr. Elvin Semrad (Adler, 1979; Zerbe, 2016, 2020, 2022a). From the 1950s until his death in 1976, Semrad was a revered educator and clinician at the Massachusetts General Hospital and Boston Psychoanalytic Institute. He used the term "tour of the body" to help psychotic patients to "go organ by organ to acknowledge and bear uncomfortable but human feelings" that they were sensing but unable to describe (Adler, 1979, p. 132). The technique can also be employed with less disturbed patients and for the clinician's own benefit (Zerbe, 2020, 2022a). While sitting with the patient or after the session, the clinician relaxes and inquires whether a particular body organ is feeling tension or discomfort that has gone unnoticed. If answered in the affirmative, the exercise can quietly unfold to a deeper level: What might this reaction be telling us? Why is it happening now? Is a painful experience or withheld secret that has no words yet being announced?

It is easy to confuse the patient's physical signals with one's own or to grasp for simple answers to dynamic constellations that are actually quite complicated. Understanding what is happening nonverbally first requires containment and the emergence of images and sensations from which interpretation gradually proceeds. To some extent, making use of the patient's and one's own embodied communication depends on the therapist's theoretical background and comfort with nonverbal, sensory stimuli.

Fortunately, a number of simple techniques beyond the unique approaches of Semrad and Sletvold can assist the therapist in assessing bodily signals. Barratt (2013) suggests that his experience as an advanced practitioner of yoga helps him focus on his own and his patient's breathing. He facetiously but accurately points out to analysts that it may be just as important to wonder "What comes to body?" as it is to ask "What comes to mind?" (2013, p. 170). The therapist's capacity to free-associate and tune in during internal states of reverie are essential entry points. Several authors have converged on the necessity to slow the pace of treatment when considering body issues (Gubb, 2014; Worrall, 2015; Zerbe, 1995, 1998, 2019, 2022a, b).

In psychoanalytic terms, Hunter's experience could be thought of as a classic case of projective identification. Audra's disavowed or unwanted mental state had mysteriously been deposited in him, and he had picked up on it because his headaches occurred only when he was with her. He wondered whether she might withholding essential information from the treatment—details they had not discussed but could potentially be perceived and accessed through another sensory mode.

While still relevant to formulating what may be happening with many different types of clinical interactions, contemporary theorists are taking a broader view. Cognitive psychology and neuroscience are enhancing our understanding: what was previously experienced as "uncanny" or "mystical" has direct application for our study of how body communications occur between people. Before delving further into some of the potential mechanisms by which this occurs, let us briefly tour the kinds of secrets routinely held by the body. These communications can be missed by therapists who are unfamiliar or uncomfortable with corporality. Unsurprisingly, excretions and sexuality—products of the body's interior realm—hold significant meaning for the clinician's next steps in the treatment.

Talking about Pleasure

Does every body hold a secret? Some days, it's more important to consider this question than others.

From discussions of a physical illness to the use of the therapist's toilet, patients describe their body as a transmitter of messages that they are not otherwise able to put into words. These communications are often obscure and messy, with answers that remain elusive because they contain shards of patients' split-off or disavowed feelings such as sadness, guilt, anger, disappointment, and rage. In Anne Power's 2016 book on retirement from clinical practice, one psychoanalyst mentions developing acute back pain after her decision to close her practice. Power observed the interviewee's struggle with retiring and wondered whether the physical pain was a way "to speak for the burden of many tangled feelings which the retiring analyst faces . . . we communicate sadness and loss through a sagging of the body" (p. 118). In this case, the retirement was openly acknowledged— that was the content behind the pain. But the feelings from which it arose were secreted in the lumbago, a psychological process that obscured the cause. Hence, this clinician maintained in silent "possession" of her actual emotions concerning retirement through physical displacement pinpointed in her lumbar muscles and spine.

The body speaks in many ways when previously unknown confidences are revealed. Gross (1951) made a compelling observation: "Emotional release affects body functions directly, particularly those of the organs of excretion, and manifests itself in a flood of tears or, perhaps the urge to urinate or defecate" (p. 39). In my practice, I have made use of the symbolic equations of a patient's need to urinate as an expression of tears; the urge to leave the session to defecate is a way to shed withheld anger or other unsavory emotions.

Keeping Gross's contribution in mind, I pose an additional question to myself: Is the patient's urgency only a mode of emotional catharsis, or has some new and complicated conflict been broached that has ignited a need to flee the room, albeit briefly? Does the patient want to rid themselves of dirtiness, shame, and rage by making a deposit in the bathroom, or does the urge signal secreted enjoyment or titillation? Excretory release can feel exciting and pleasurable. At the revelatory moment of exit from the office, neither patient nor therapist can know what gratifications might have been unlocked.

The gendered body holds further secrets, some of them sexually alluring. The body ego of females is shaped by the interior sexual organs that promotes a girl's development of fantasy life and the capacity for reverie and solitude. Interiority also enables females to keep an entire range of pleasurable body sensations secret, adding a sense of mystery and "power in the ability to keep a secret and to choose to share it or not" (Kulish, 2002, p. 156). Clinicians may overlook the enjoyment and excitement associated with sexual arousal because of unconscious conflict by either member of the dyad. Physical pleasure in the past, present, and future remains the patient's secret!

Balsam (2015) pointed out that Freud was positive and curious about his famous patient Dora's open, robust sexual yearnings but backed away from helping her constructively deal with them in the treatment because of rigid sexual mores in nineteenth-century European society. His cultural countertransference thwarted Dora's opportunity to elaborate her desire and personal narrative, stifling development of self. Dora eventually fled the analysis (Freud, 1905).[1]

Even though Western society appears to be less conflicted about robust expressions of pleasure for both men and women, contemporary clinicians may likewise be prone to neglect inquiries about the body and sexuality— and the secret stories they hold. Therapists tend to embrace a métier as primarily healers of people's pain. It's important to remember that the body may be harboring its pleasurable secrets too, and our patients may need considerable prompting to tell us what feels good as well as bad. The interactive nature of contemporary psychotherapeutic technique catalyzes a process in which "the aim and focus of action in therapy are not simply to divine the content of a secret but, more importantly, the process of sharing it" (Kulish, 2002, p. 171).

Emboldened after rereading Michigan Training Analyst Nancy Kulish's paper, I found myself wondering whether a spry, elderly widower who had undergone full resection of the prostate for cancer over a decade prior was still sexually active. Self-supervision alerted me to consider that this patient and I were colluding in a cocreated resistance (Samberg, 2004). I decided to inquire. He gleefully replied, "Of course! Medical science provides us fellows with lots of bells and whistles. I've been waiting for you to ask!"

Working with Somatic Countertransference Reactions

Somatic (or embodied) countertransference reactions are a kind of signal to the therapist that the patient harbors hidden knowledge that cannot be revealed in words. Appreciating somatic countertransference builds on acceptance of the role of the body as communicator of sometimes unspeakable feelings and storylines. Unrecognized physical effects accumulate for therapists over the course of careers spent absorbing so much of what patients deem unacceptable or disturbing. Sometimes a session or series of sessions may prove quite illuminating. Hunter's observation that his headaches communicated an unspoken factor blocking the treatment led him to propose that he and Audra pursue historical facts not previously elaborated.

Somatic countertransference includes a wide swath of embodied information that the clinician perceives within a given patient-therapist encounter (Field, 1988; Gubb, 2014; Worrall, 2015; Zerbe, 2022a, b). Any sensory or physiologic system can be employed to send the clandestine message. Body sensations are therefore one source of information that can help guide the treatment but require ongoing self-analysis like Hunter Allen undertook.

This reflective process helps the therapist avoid making assumptions and defaulting to self-referentiality. After all, the therapist's feelings or emotional state do not always convey something about the patient that should be commented on or interpreted. Applying somatic countertransference to a clinical case formulation requires judicious self-scrutiny in conjunction with other sources of clinical data (Abassi, 2018; Allen, 2013) and implies a specific somatosensory response that differs from other forms of body attunement, such as nonverbal resonance, musicality, synchronous vocalization, and the emotional background of the session (Blum, Goldberg, & Levin, 2023; Knoblauch, 2000, 2005, 2011; Markman, 2020, 2022; Wilson, 2018).

After decades of research in cognitive neuroscience, Wilma Bucci concluded that mammals use a variety of codes to communicate with each other and to process that information (Bucci, 1997, 2008, 2011a, b; Bucci & Cornell, 2021). Subsymbolic systems documented in fMRI and TMS studies "operating without explicit intention or direction . . . [that] occur in specific sensory-somatic modalities . . . [underlie] the analyst's sensing of the patient's inner states" (Bucci & Cornell, 2021, p. 32).

Science now has a refined explanation for what may be experienced as uncanny, intuitive, or mystical, so Bucci prefers that clinicians avoid terms like "projective identification" and "the analytic third." Instead, she uses the apt metaphor of an invisible umbilical cord that is always operative and links individuals in relationships (Bucci, 2018). Emotional processing in subsymbolic formats occurs continuously and wordlessly and is ultimately responsible for what clinicians subsume under the rubric of "empathy, intuition, and unconscious communication . . . Language has been assumed to be the primary medium of psychoanalysis (the 'talking cure') although it is not the primary medium of thought and certainly not emotion" (p. 33). Ironically, embodied communication and the mutuality of its expression are not wallflowers at the dance; rather, they initiate it.

The Stories We Tell: A Documentary Film about Family Secrets

Director, author, and actor Sarah Polley has been a household name in Canada since her youth. A child star in many highly successful Canadian television programs, her international acclaim continues to expand across media.[2] Her autobiographical documentary *Stories We Tell* (2012) captures one individual gradually facing and disentangling a disconcerting family secret that overshadowed her life.

The movie exemplifies what in my practice I call a "not-known known." When all the pieces of a concealed aspect of family history are pulled together and clarified, it turns out few individuals affected by the revelation are actually surprised. "I knew it all the time! I just didn't know that

I knew."[3] To reveal and gain personal peace, or to continue on in order to protect the status quo? That's the conundrum.

Prior to unraveling and disclosing an oppressive secret, people can feel ashamed or even question their sanity when, in fact, they've been imprisoned in a long-standing double bind. Despite the hidden history, it's not unusual for these patients I've treated to have sensed subtleties of others' communications. Often other family members held a key to the puzzle, and patients suffered considerable worry around unveiled secrets overturning the equilibrium among loved ones.

I usually recommend the film *Stories We Tell* to clinicians like Hunter, as well as to certain patients struggling with destructive secrets. Shared reference points from the film expand the therapeutic conversation. It's a rich human story that leaves the viewer feeling less alone and more tolerant of the layers of confusing messages they continue to feel forced to "not know and know" simultaneously. At a crossroads, how does one decide whether to further a quest for details or to leave well enough alone?

Director Polley combines interviews in real time, directing actors playing her parents and their friends in film clips made to look vintage; their script is taken from her father's memoir and narrated by him. The result is a deep dive that initially resolves mysteries surrounding her mother Diane, who died when Polley was eleven years old. It eventuates in her discovery that her biological father was different from the man who raised her. Each person entwined in this enigmatic world has their own take on what actually transpired in Diane's life. From within the close family nexus of father and four siblings, the revelation ripples outward to friends and colleagues of Diane who come to share what they knew, or assumed they knew, about Polley's actual parentage.

How did people think they knew the secret story of Polley's real father? The child's physical appearance apparently held an important clue about the mystery. Until her death, Polley's mother repeatedly commented on her daughter's unusual red hair. Did that awaken suspicion in others? Growing up, Sarah recalls being teased by her older brother because she didn't look like any of her other siblings.

As the film unfolds, this brother recollects overhearing their mother, Diane, murmur on the phone to someone that she became pregnant during an affair. Throughout the film, viewers hear assumptions and fantasies from other family and friends who guessed the identity of her biological father. While some interviewees managed to keep what they suspected inviolate even as the camera rolled, others were more candid and let down their guard, revealing their suppositions to the writer-director.

Through Polley's creative process, the viewer sees that every individual might have their own self-told truths, but these facts are not immutable. Newly discovered information invites some people to take a second look.

Of course, others double down on the old truth, but what we believe about ourselves and our loved ones is more fluid than we know. Reassessment has the power to reconfigure self-knowledge and sometimes change the course of life.

While some may claim the right to own the official story of another person, each of us is left to transmogrify whatever residual impingement lingers on our own psyche and soma from others' narratives. The candor with which Polley addresses her embodied secret has been helpful to some of my patients and, I assume, to millions of others. Hence, I think of her contribution through the medium of film as a gift for the greater good—the psychological well-being of society.

The journey of discovery that Polley depicts was bound to change her life's course. Other spoken messages, or more subtle clues she received from those close to her, might parallel what patients face in similar circumstances. But how can we apply lessons from Polley's discerning lens in our consulting room? Additional insights from neuropsychology and contemporary biology can be used to help patients appreciate that a "not-known known" has physiological bases that simultaneously ground their own perceptions and catalyze the process of bringing stultifying secrets into the open.

The Possible Role of Mirror Neurons

How, in fact, do we know what we don't know? The late twentieth-century discovery of the mirror neuron system may explain the mechanics of the intersubjective connection forged between human beings. When a therapist is bedeviled by an impasse and senses a patient is not saying everything, it is highly conceivable that interlinked mirror neuron systems are doing their job. In essence, a message is verbally withheld but nonverbally communicated from the patient to the therapist through complex neural networks and subsymbolic communication pathways. Mirror neurons are what make this possible.

This interlinked system could undergird new hypotheses about how, why, and under what conditions secrets are maintained—and sometimes courageously released—within intimate human relationships. As neuroscience has consistently demonstrated, individuals who are engaged with each other have a built-in and involuntary capacity to simulate emotional experience in others (Cozolino, 2017; Gallese, 2006, 2011; Ginot, 1997, 2009, 2015; Vivona, 2009a, b). Over eons, the mirror neuron system has evolved within us to send implicit information back and forth between people physically close to each other in a fraction of a microsecond.

While the mirror neurons pick up signals and nonverbal messaging, it's obvious that they can only go so far in what they convey. They don't expose precise content, but they let us know something important is going on with another person or persons in our environment. In Chapter 3, Michael experienced a "fog" that cleared after he learned about his father's other family. The entwined mirror neuron system between him and his father could be one explanation for the evaporating mental haze that occurred after his father finally told Michael the truth. Through nonconscious communication, Michael automatically tuned in to his father's unspoken secret. The emotional and communicational impermeability between them dissipated after the truth was spoken aloud.

The mirror neuron system enables individuals to maintain a sense of self while viscerally and empathically "observing and imitating" connections (Ginot, 2015, p. 90) with other people. It sends signals to the limbic system through the anterior insula and is especially active in the parietal and frontal lobes of the right hemisphere establishing "a neuropsychological link between interacting subjectivities that observe and relate to each other" (p. 113). These "neurologically linked subjectivities" suggest that keeping a secret may be more conspicuous than we assume, especially to those with whom we live in close proximity or to whom we have an emotional tether (Akhtar, 1992).

Loyal sons like Michael feel enormous relief when an important attachment relationship remains unbroken after they address the unspoken— once they are permitted to "know" what their mirror neurons have intersubjectively been telling them for a long time. The fog cleared because Michael and his father could start forging a space to dialogue openly and interpersonally. On the neurophysiological level, myriad mirror neuron networks had always connected the two individuals. Hence, Michael's embodied sense of living in a cloud of bewilderment persisted until the clarifying words broke through.

The mirror neuron system supposedly mediates emotions in subcortical and cortical regions via links to the amygdala, particularly in the right brain. That would mean that fear responses could readily arise at the mere utterance of a furtive story—all in service of protecting an essential relationship. One might also wonder whether certain patients have an extraordinary manifestation of fear conditioning derived from reinforced connectivity of the amygdala and mirror neuron system. The munificent layering of neural networks reifies the propensity to inhibit expression of narrative, fantasy, and emotional experiences. For these individuals, the intimate and private is hijacked by complex neural networks at the expense of higher cortical functions and autobiographical synthesis.

While there is as yet no way to know precisely which neural circuits are responsible for maintaining secrets on the borderlands of conscious-unconscious phenomena, the evolutionarily early, primitive, fast-acting fear system must be overridden by the later-evolving, slower prefrontal cortex (Ginot, 2015; Panksepp, 2009; Panksepp & Biven, 2012) for certain truths to be shared. Clinicians who assist patients in discovering and working through unconscious loyalty oaths made within family systems may help reset these automatic functions of the brain. What they are doing is providing a safe haven in which anxiety-ridden self-states need no longer be on automatic pilot.

A Lesson from Stacy

When I speak at conferences about the bodily impact of withholding important truths, I always honor other secret-keeping professions, such as clergy, attorneys, inventors, intelligence officers, law enforcement personnel, journalists, and military brass. In fact, one of my presentation slides names some of these occupations, a prompt to get people thinking about the many careers that include elements of preserving confidences. I remind the audience members that the particular ethical standards regarding disclosure and confidentiality that bind each profession may become part of the therapeutic conversation.

In psychotherapy, private facts about others associated with the patient's career may be deliberately shared or inadvertently revealed. It's the psychotherapist's responsibility to help the patient to acknowledge and evaluate what is ethically mandated by their professional role that may also burden their psyche and soma. Those of us who make our living listening are often surprised by how routinely patients describe aspects of their work that they must be tight-lipped about—but that they also intuitively sense influences their well-being. Perhaps when a patient divulges covert pressures their occupation creates, they are asking for permission to take the consequences seriously and begin to ameliorate these underappreciated, subliminally sensed deleterious consequences. Just as I observed in the psychotherapy consultation of Hunter Allen, individuals in all secret-keeping fields may be paying a heavier price for what they do than they are consciously aware.

In lectures I ask the audience, "Is there a noteworthy secret-keeping profession deliberately left off this list? What is it?" Without a moment's hesitation, women clinicians raise their arms and shout out in unison: "Hairstylists!"

I've been curious since I was a teenager about how hairdressers listen to their clients tell story after story, some of them quite personal and revealing, and wondered what they do with the information at the end of the day. Do they take the stories home with them? Do they worry about some of them? What happens when a favorite client known for years has a vexing family issue or life-threatening health problem? Do braggarts spark jealousy or envy? Or stir up a stylist's buried trauma or secrets? And how do they manage everyday slights and complaints? Have they found ways to grow thick skin because they realize some people can never be pleased? Do stylists gossip these beauty parlor secrets to family or friends?

Psychotherapists are routinely asked similar questions about our careers by friends and family members. My long-standing curiosity about and questioning of hairstylists serves a dual purpose. I thirst for more knowledge about how confidences emerge and are kept in professional relationships, and I search just as hard for clues and tips in general about how kindred professionals manage common stressors that arise from holding off-the-record information. Because of comparison points to psychoanalytic training institutes, I'm especially curious how stylists in small towns or communities manage the intriguing, puzzling news and gossip that comes their way. Does the response depend on who the client is? Or the social situation the stylist finds himself in? Some innuendos may be heard repeatedly, but with different nuances that stir up feelings. This parallels the dilemma of psychotherapists and psychoanalysts, who must learn to manage what is rumored or known about others in our personal and professional communities.

While a hairstylist doesn't have the same ethical duty as a therapist to keep confidentiality, the listener's role and many of the challenges cross disciplines in terms of both rewards and hazards. If a stylist violates trust, a client might quit. When a stylist hears a heartbreaking tale, they can't pick up and go home in the middle of the day if there's a full slate of appointments on the books. Business depends on dependability, steadiness, and tact. The intimate human bond with clients often grows over the years but can be easily severed when a client moves, dies, or simply stops coming.

So, in what ways is a hairstylist's job like a psychotherapist? Both must maintain boundaries, but they aren't spelled out by a clear ethical code for the stylist as they are for the therapist. A stylist might feel burdened by what they learn about other people, especially personal information. Life stories that a stylist hears about, and then must process, could lodge in their body as much as the cumulative effect from all the digital manipulations, arm lifting, leg pumping, standing, cutting, turning, and position shifting required in their role but taken as "just a part of the job." What methods have they found for taking care of themselves?

I've put my curiosity to a test. What do hairdressers do with all the personal data they take in from their clients and how do they metabolize it? Since I've been asking the questions in some form or other since my teens and gotten roughly the same answers, I decided to more formally interview a dozen or so additional stylists for fun while writing this book. While the precise language and particular questions I use evolved over the years, the inquiry has always gone something like this:

> People must tell you all kinds of interesting things about their lives. What's it like to hear peoples' stories all day long.
>
> If someone tells you something and says that it's private and you can't tell anyone else, do you find you can keep it to yourself?
>
> Does it ever drive you a little batty? Or can you usually let it go and put it out of your mind at the end of the appointment?
>
> Have you ever found yourself circling back to a particular story or difficult situation that a client is struggling with after work? What do you do if this happens?

The consistency in answers is remarkable. The overwhelming majority of stylists tell me that they enjoy hearing others' stories but are only rarely affected by what they hear. In fact, one stylist I interviewed for this book said,

> Frankly, it goes in one ear and out the other. I tell the client they can 'tell me anything and it will stay right here.' I mean it. I don't make a point of dwelling on the details. I'm too busy with my own life when I get home.

In general, hairstylists tell me how much they enjoy their profession and the mutual interaction that is an essential part of their job, and they don't feel a particular obligation to offer guidance or advice. Many let me in on a professional secret and hoped I would not take offense: "Do you know they start telling us in beauty school to get ready to hear all kinds of issues people have because we're 'kind of like therapists' in our job?" Some acknowledged that they offer encouragement (or what I translate as empathy) when a client discusses a problem. All but one told me that they knew they were privy to personal information but sensed no physical or psychological burden when listening.

There were, however, two notable exceptions to the unperturbed chorus. One woman in her late twenties explained that she was in the process of studying to become a paralegal at a community college; she enjoyed cosmetology school but found the ongoing human element of hearing problems as a stylist "something that drags me down. I don't have the life experience to offer counsel. It gets me off-kilter and I lose my focus on the hair." She looked forward to joining a legal firm where she could spend most days quietly doing research alone.

In another situation, a salon owner told me that a husband and wife both regularly had their hair done at her establishment for years.

The husband was a transvestite in his seventies. The wife made the couple's appointments to get their monthly trims. However, she also set up a separate monthly appointment for her husband. For that appointment, he is booked under the name Maude, his female persona. Maude arrived beautifully attired in gowns to get her wigs coifed. The stylist told me she felt it was a privilege to be trusted by the couple with this shared knowledge and did not feel burdened by it whatsoever. However, as we spoke together in the interview, she registered considerable relief by telling someone who lived out of town and couldn't "blab." She had protected the couple's truth even from her closest confidants: "I've never let it slip to my dear husband, who can be quite judgmental about such matters."

Several hairstylists rattled off heartbreaking tales of colleagues they knew who had to quit their profession because of physical tolls such as arthritis, orthopedic issues in their arms, legs, or feet, and chronic back pain or spine deterioration. But only rarely did a client's confession leave a stylist with little left to fully attend to family or friends at the end of a long day. Was it possible that all the information simply went in one ear and out the other? They recognized the bona fide physical costs of the job that add up over years but denied that what they heard about the lives of others had any effect on their body whatsoever. It didn't fit with what most therapists experience about our work and the necessary awareness in both professions about ongoing self-care needs.

I've turned the discrepancy over in my mind repeatedly for years. Were the stylists in denial? Could it be that they were out of touch with this aspect of embodiment when they heard so many details about the lives of others? Could it be that they just didn't feel comfortable saying more to a probing psychiatrist? One day, I confided this dilemma to my hairstylist Stacy Morin (personal communication, 2021) and told her that I simply did not find the dismissals of the interviewees believable whatsoever.

Stacy retorted, "Oh, I find it highly believable, Kassy. Everyone you talked to was telling you their version of the truth."

"How do you do it then, Stacy? It's simply impossible. Listen all day and not let it affect you?"

Stacy stopped momentarily, put her scissors down, and turned her attention inward. I sensed she already knew her answer and paused to figure out just how she would make her point.

"Because I am not *just* listening."

She then rested her hands on my shoulders and asked me to look straight into the mirror. She continued to explain: "When someone is in my chair getting their hair done, my eyes and hands continually focus on their face. I must be sure the cut is even—what we call 'balance'—or that the color treatment is turning out the precise shade I'm aiming to achieve.

"Every client is different. Attention is paid to detail, especially at the end when I texturize. You can always trim more but as we say in the trade, 'when it's gone, it's gone.'"

Noticing my perplexity, Stacy took her hands off my shoulders and stepped backward.

She suddenly put her foot on the pedal of her styling chair and quickly raised me off the ground another six inches. She stepped back and walked from side to side a few times, all the while keeping one eye peeled on my head, another skirting the periphery of my torso. I understood that she was exaggerating her "hairstylist pose" for effect to teach me something important about her experience.

She continued. "See what I'm doing? Look closer. I move back and forth and around every client multiple times to be sure that I am getting things just the way I want. I check to see if they're satisfied. So, I do tune in and pay attention to what is being said that's personal, but my job is doing their hair. That takes most of my time, energy, and attention during the appointment.

"After a person has been a regular client for months, you know their hair so you can be more social. But I never forget that my primary job is always doing their hair."

Talk about the value of field research! A stylist instinctively moves while keeping the primary focus on the job at hand. Moving is also essential to their work. A sedentary therapist, however, must remember to grab opportunities in between sessions to recharge physically and psychologically and is challenged to claim this space given multiple demands to return calls, finish notes and billing, and keep pace with the schedule.

Stacy was demonstrating in vivo a lesson from the neurology textbooks: the value of selective attention in consciousness. Selective attention is the capacity grounded in neurobiological evolution that guides and sharpens our neural machinery, depending upon what we do. Information processing by our brain is regulated by major neuromodulatory systems—cholinergic, serotoninergic, noradrenergic pathways—that enable mammals to attend to one subject in the external world to the exclusion of others (Giuliano, Karns, Bell, Petersen, et al., 2018; Kandel, Koester, Mack, & Siegelbaum, 2022; Lane & Pearson, 1982; Plude, Enns, & Brodeur, 1994; Van Gerven & Guerreiro, 2016)

Throughout the course of life, our neural networks are continually modified by experience. In the case of a hairstylist, the work requires exquisite development and ongoing coordination of fine motor skills, the visual system, and sensorimotor pathways—that is, touch. The parietal cortex makes connections to the prefrontal areas of the brain so that delicate movement of the eyes and hands synchronize with upper- and lower-body musculature (Eagleman, 2020; Kandel et al., 2022). Because the hairstylist is using so many parts of the body at every moment, and not *just* their listening skills, they are exercising a natural, built-in defense against the deleterious effects that one absorbs when exclusively focusing on hearing, remembering, and staying mum about what may be confided.

As Stacy says, she listens, but she does not *just* listen. Cortical maps modify based on what is used and not used, and selective attention relies upon this property of the brain's inherent plasticity. These operations likely serve a protective function for professions in which there is a significant degree of physicality involved. Hearing stories and personal details of another's life are "worked out" by all the different kinds of body motions that Stacy described. They are not attended to exclusively because the brain is paying better attention to something else. The color, shape, texture, and balance of the hairstyle take precedence, along with all the notable but unconscious physical prowess cultivated in cosmetology school and over years of practice in doing the job.

Stacy's story drives home another important lesson from twenty-first-century neurobiology that is vital for all of us to keep in mind: Everything we do—including listening—takes energy! Our body is continually budgeting for the demands that our environment places on us. An ample body budget enables us to attend to others while continually tuning, pruning, and rewiring our neural networks in our ever-changing world (Barrett, 2020; Barrett & Finlay, 2018; Barrett & Quigley, 2021). Hairdressers and therapists occupy different social and environmental niches that require different tools, fine-tuning our brains to details, and unconsciously parceling our body budget to effectively work with the techniques of our craft. Neuroscientist Lisa Feldman Barratt (2020) makes an eloquent analogy to the brain's evolutionary ability to selectively attend to information, and then rewire and achieve the focus required of human endeavors:

> (It's) similar to a spotlight in the darkness. . . . your brain network contains smaller communities of neurons whose main job is to focus on certain details as important and ignore other details as irrelevant. Your brain focuses its spotlight of attention continually and automatically, and often you're unaware that it's happening . . . If you constantly struggle in a simmering sea of stress, and your body budget accrues an ever-deepening deficit, that's called chronic stress . . . (and) can gradually eat away at your brain and cause illness in your body.
>
> (p. 91)

Hearing another person's secret throws a spotlight on what was shrouded in darkness, revising our picture of that individual's narrative just as much as it does for the teller, whose tale is now exposed. But we must remember that it inevitably also draws from the attuned listener's account of even the most plentiful body budget. Being "all ears" over hours and days can tax our body, particularly when we are going through a rough patch in our own life.

Good listeners and confidence keepers have always been well advised to take time to refuel, reflect, and refresh because of the sheer amount of discreet information that is entrusted to us and absorbed by us. Now we know that it's a biological necessity. Shakespeare's aphorism "Self-love, my liege, is not so vile a sin as self-neglecting" is a powerful yet a gentle reminder to those who tend to the needs of others. Find time and space to tend also to yourself.

We all must cultivate an individualized skill set to make regular deposits into our own body budget account: pausing, relaxing, reading, getting consultation, nurturing friendships, pursuing hobbies. A good listener positively impacts the body budget of anyone who becomes less burdened and relieved of stress because they talked it out. It's a humanistic perspective that neuroscientist Barrett echoes when she observes the basic biological benefit derived from intersubjectivity and interdependence in relationships, wherein

Each of us can be the kind of person who makes more deposits into other people's body budgets than withdrawals. . . . Your brain secretly works with other brains. This hidden cooperation keeps us healthy, so it matters how we treat one another in a very real, brain-wiring way.

(p. 97)

Mirror neurons help us balance not only our own body budgets but also those of our patients and everyone we interact with.

Talk, Walk, and Write

When I've presented Stacy's hairstyling insight at conferences, participants ask what they can do to take care of themselves. The question itself lets me know they've gotten the message.

Secrets are ubiquitous in our line of work. We pick up on them even when they are not yet fully conscious to us or to those in our care. Working with such radioactive material has significant impact on the psychological and physical well-being of our patients as well as ourselves. Some microtraumas and impasses are predictable, as Hunter Allen experienced. Is there anything short of lifelong psychotherapy—or totally ditching the work we love—to render us immune to the somatic ill effects of taking in so many disturbing and often painful histories?

I've developed a simple mnemonic for clinician well-being. It is based on all the research data, qualitative studies, psychodynamic concepts, and clinical stories I cover in this book.

Here's the short version: Talk, walk, and write!

Each element is aimed at helping clinicians remember that we can do something quite simple, but vastly important, to mitigate secrecy's wear and tear on us. Hardworking therapists are at substantially elevated risk for burnout. We must acknowledge the cumulative toll of the secrets we become privy to in our profession. Paying attention to our ongoing self-care needs and practicing the three steps require time, attention, and commitment. Nonetheless, as the data show, consistency pays off handsomely.

Talk. While those in the secret-keeping professions don't need to be in lifelong therapy ourselves, each of us can benefit from someone with whom to consistently talk and process disturbing information in a confidential setting. Oftentimes, that person is a supervisor or a consultant. This can occur in an individual or group setting and does not have to be a continuous process. Sometimes, it works to have just a few sessions with someone who has a different point of view or to attend a conference that includes time for small-group processing of clinical work. Many clinicians enjoy and learn from established, regular meetings with like-minded and trusted peers.

Walk. Clinicians need to stay grounded through physical activity to restore the body budget, to exercise across modal neurophysiological systems so that information is distributed, and to enhance these feedback mechanisms. I use the word "walk" as a rhyming memory prompt to stay mindful of the body's need to move. Yoga, Pilates, strength training, team sports, or the research-based advice to have several "exercise snacks" in a day—meaning taking several short five-minute breaks of physical activity each day—can serve the purpose. One need not run a marathon to go the distance of having a long career as a sedentary therapist. Benefits of keeping the body active and grounded accrue over time.

Write. Find a place to write down the troubling or traumatic stories you hear. You don't necessarily need to keep a journal. A few notes or lists will help you process what you have taken in during the day or week. There may be some advantage accrued by handwriting as opposed to typing on computer (James & Engelhardt, 2012; Mueller & Oppenheimer, 2014). Whatever method works for you will suffice. The notes can then be shredded, deleted, or filed away, depending on your preference and professional guidelines. Should you feel a little silly when jotting, pause to reconsider the robust health benefits of the studies Pennebaker undertook of students who wrote about their traumatic experiences (see Chapter 3).

Conclusion

Secrets that have not been previously revealed in psychotherapy may be first noticed by a somatic (or embodied) countertransference reaction.

These corporeal experiences are defined as occurring within a specific therapist-patient dyad and occur more frequently than either party is aware. These intersubjective signals are easily dismissed because they can fluster and or unnerve the therapist. Somatic countertransference is as important to appreciate and understand as any other countertransference experience but has not received the attention it deserves in clinical training or in the literature.

The body's countertransference cues may be as subtle as a twinge in the neck or an urge to urinate, or they may be as intrusive as a headache or as loud as intestinal noises. These reactions are essential to decode because they are a point of access into the patient's tangled web of feelings and to the unspoken storyline routinely split off from conscious awareness. Somatic countertransference must be integrated with other strands of clinical data and differentiated from the therapist's idiosyncratic feelings that arise in treatment. To become more conversant with their body and attuned to what the patient's body might be nonverbally communicating, clinicians can practice a number of relatively easy techniques.

Fortunately, embodied reactivity that occurs in the therapeutic dyad is receiving renewed and exciting attention in psychotherapy. Cognitive neuroscience and medical research are at the forefront in promoting ways of understanding once lumped under the rubric of the intuitive, uncanny, or mystical feeling states that occur between a therapist and a patient. Multiple biological pathways are involved every time a clinician picks up on any intersubjective communications, and additional complex mechanisms of action will surely be discovered in the future. Subsymbolic communications, mirror neurons, body budgeting, and selective attention are included in the clinical formulations of this chapter because they form a credible foundation for understanding the paradoxical and mystifying state of simultaneously knowing and not knowing a secret.

However, some authorities argue that an appreciation of these cognitive and neurobiological perspectives is unnecessary for—and may even hamper—deeper, expressive therapeutic work. They point out that a medical explanation never satisfies a person in emotional distress. This has not been my experience, particularly when it comes to patients who must grapple with a withheld family secret—or a "not-known known" in their lives. Actually, some patients are relieved to learn ways they may have attuned to others' injunctions through brain-based mechanisms such as the mirror neuron system or subsymbolic communication channels. That information makes them feel more human, less flummoxed, and, to some extent, emboldened to take next steps in their therapeutic journey. In effect, education empowers by helping the patient appreciate how their brain was simply doing its job: picking up on multiple, competing, and divergent signals and expending exhaustive amounts of energy to do so.

Health-wise, it is as important for the clinician as it is for the patient to be mindful of these neurocognitive and biological findings. In the therapeutic cauldron, the therapist is continually exposed to receiving and sending embodied communications. Safeguarding confidential information, listening, and containing secrets all have additional impact on the body budget, making ongoing self-care imperative. Based on all the research data, qualitative studies, psychodynamic concepts, and clinical examples described thus far in this book, the mnemonic "Talk, Walk, and Write" guides clinicians to body-mind wellness in the face of intense secret-keeping demands.

Notes

1 Late in life, Freud helped his eighteen-year-old patient Margarethe Walter claim a sense of autonomy and pleasure. Margarethe's father refused to listen to her career aspirations and forbade her to watch kissing scenes when they went to the movies together. In this restrictive environment, her father forced Freud to take the history while sitting between himself and his daughter. (Afterward, Freud insisted upon private interviews.) Margarethe then disclosed a secret to Freud. She told him she "would devour spicy, titillating books" (Loewenberg, 2017, p. 665) tucked away in the grown-ups' locked bookshelves. She read privately at night when the family was asleep, her healthy sexual appetite obviously implied. As Freud listened, he also discovered that Margarethe had career aspirations of her own. Instead of assuming the successful family business as expected, she wanted to become a sculptress. Mortified by the intrusions that obstructed his patient's burgeoning sense of self, Freud "sternly prescribed" that she embrace adulthood, stay in her seat at the movies and watch kissing scenes, and remember what Freud told her if she withered. At age eighty-eight, this former patient, who became a noted Austrian sculptress, was interviewed. She told cultural writer Peter Roos that the forty-five-minute session with Freud changed her life (Slavin & Rahmani, 2016). Margarethe Walter Lutz commented on Freud's "unbelievable attentiveness," which unlocked a body-based feeling of contentment, "like having an especially good meal, and on top of that as if someone had opened the window and said: 'Don't always look at the floor! Look outside! All is possible.'" (Loewenberg, p. 666).

2 Sarah Polley is perhaps best known for writing and directing the Academy Award–winning movie *Women Talking* (2022). In this film and in her collection of autobiographical essays *Run toward the Danger: Confrontations with a Body of Memory* (2022), individuals come to grips with the "not known knowns" in their lives. The previously unspeakable but obvious concealment of sexual trauma and boundary violation to multiple women is painstakingly recounted and eventually faced. The essays suggest the impact of pernicious secret keeping on psyche and body of this kind, which I discuss in the book; the movie explicitly depicts the crimes and blows of religious indoctrination that enabled generational submission of women, eventually quietly voiced by a courageous few in the presence of their scribe, a supportive male witness.

3 For clinical examples of not known knowns, see K. Zerbe (2019), "The Secret Life of Secrets: Deleterious Psychosomatic Effects on Patient and Analyst," *Journal of the American Psychoanalytic Association,* 67, 185—214. In one remarkable case, an adolescent girl supposedly had no awareness that she was

conceived by sperm donation through an in vitro fertilization process. She was obsessed with a repetitive auditory hallucination: "Don't say it. Don't Say it." This psychotic symptom subsided when she was finally given permission to speak about what she knew. It remained unclear in the treatment if the child had subliminally or overtly overheard members of her family talk about the actual circumstances of the conception or if this parcel of information had been intersubjectively communicated. Either way, the precocious patient got the message about what she should not say and loyally complied until the clinicians working with her and her family prevailed to make the previously unspeakable speakable.

6 The Complicated Ethics of Concealment

My friend Claire Morgan thumbed through the torn leather album until she found her favorite wedding photograph. Out of the corner of her eye, she detected that I was curious to hear more about the teenage girls pictured in front of the Grenada Theatre on an earlier page. Quickly changing topic from the ruddy-complexioned Marine lieutenant she divorced ten years before we met, Claire began to enlighten me about the snapshot and growing up African American in a small college town southeast of Chicago.

"We always knew the best seats in the house were in the balcony when we were little. Not being *allowed* to sit in the orchestra was the horrible irony. Became a great place to make out with guys by our teens—our own secluded 'den of iniquity,'" she chuckled.

I counted on Claire for the unvarnished truth. I wasn't the only one. By her middle years, an assortment of diverse women inevitably lined up for advice or solace outside her university office. As director of the student learning center and minority liaison to the associate dean, she found herself sorting through undergraduate and faculty grievances and requests for assistance and advice. The scope of our careers as listeners and secret keepers overlapped in oddly similar ways. We would get together for supper every month or so for what we called mutual brain-combing sessions.

I'd get to hear the latest bon mots she doled out to her underlings, appropriating them as needed for my developing career. I once laughed and told her, "Help the world by hanging out your own counseling shingle! You'd put us shrinks out of business. I don't get why you spend your days sifting through administrative red tape and writing boring policy memos. You'd earn more, Claire!"

She retorted, "And I don't get why you shrinks don't get that nobody arrives any too cheerful to see you. Have you considered the cost?"

DOI: 10.4324/9781003471578-7

The thing is that Claire couldn't tell a lie—not even a harmless one, and even when it would likely be for her own good. Her penchant for pointed maxims always piqued my envy:

- Should you find yourself talking with a parent whose baby isn't particularly cute, say, "I always forget how tiny and delicate they are."
- Be careful when you give a false compliment. Someone might believe the carrot-anchovy cheese dip is really your favorite appetizer.
- If a friend or relative is complaining because they're not dating yet after a bad breakup, it's time to remind them, "Everyone thinks to be truly happy you need someone in your life to make you miserable."

A couple of times Claire and I invited our buddy Charles to join us at a favorite jazz haunt for happy hour. That is, until he proposed discreet ménage-à-trois afterward. Claire snickered at the transgressive invitation and shifted into sarcastic mode. "Sure . . . like I'm craving that syrupy Madeira port they gave us to sample last month? I'll skip the tasting menu, thank you."

Claire was preternaturally disposed to impartiality and avoided judging others' choices. I assumed that the trait was so ingrained because of all the racial disparities she experienced growing up, and I struggled to speak my mind about this perception without offending. Claire's gifts still irked me sometimes. She could stop midway through a tightly reasoned opinion and reverse herself, especially when we were on the same page. I relished her trenchant point of view but knew her capacity for empathic listening could run its course. When she had her fill of anyone's failure to take responsibility for themselves, she chided, "I'm sure you've done all you can. You simply need to sound off to me!"

This attribute of fundamental fairness remained even when we talked about her deceiving ex-husband. One evening during brain combing, Claire confided,

> As you might imagine, when Russ was stationed in Shreveport in the 1960s, we were quite the item. I'll always appreciate how he tried to think about what it might be like to live in my body—in my skin—especially when we walked downtown and got evil eyes. Those glares sickened me. I tried to hide my feelings. Once I had to turn away from four men saluting some Confederate soldiers' statues on the square. Russ felt my arm get steely cold and my fingernails dig into his starched shirt. He said, 'Claire, you just don't see color. But their poison darts pierce and the toxin seeps in and scramble your system anyway. Someday those four dudes might realize they lost the war!'

Gobsmacked, I realized Claire's power to absorb and reconfigure was an unconsciously refined fortification, corporally strengthened throughout childhood and unyielding in adulthood to subvert incoming trauma. Her stealth foreswore an allergy to praise except from hopeful new mothers who bore witness to how she could "soothe even the most cantankerous baby."

The Therapist's Camouflage

Clinicians cultivate modes of concealment to help guard the secrets of others. We typically ignore the disguises and masks we wear in professional life, but, over time, they raise ethical and personal conflicts that may play havoc with our sense of identity—the very foundation of who we think we are as human beings.

Pulitzer Prize–winning journalist Lucinda Franks, whose father was an espionage agent during World War II, speaks to the insidious and largely unconscious price paid by individuals and their family members who cultivate the skills to subtly shift self-states in her memoir *My Father's Secret War* (2007). Considering the many long-term impacts of her father's secret keeping, she observes, "All those hobbies he'd thrown himself into—expert astronomer, marksman, lepidopterist—were those just different kinds of camouflage? If you have to play a part all the time, do you lose touch with who you really are?" (p. 156).

Franks's memoir serves as a cautionary tale for clinicians, which we will return to at the end of this chapter. While practicing psychotherapy does not expose one to the degree of horrors, ethical decisions, or layers of deception required of a spy or federal agent, there are parallels that raise essential questions about the personal challenges inherent in certain professions like psychotherapy. Becoming conversant with such hazards equips the therapist to maintain necessary self-care while attending to the needs of patients.

What defenses must a secret keeper cultivate to do their job well? When do professional adaptations become problematic? Can loved ones be harmed by professional camouflage? In these concerns, the tradecraft of an espionage agent and a therapist converges to an extent that any differences are of degree than of kind. In both professions, one becomes adept in the art of evasion and full expression of self.

Because therapists maintain confidentiality as part of our professional obligation, we learn to dodge questions or even obfuscate in some situations we encounter. While encouraged to share "with strictest discretion" (Freud, 1940, p. 173) private information about the patient with a supervisor or consultant to facilitate the treatment, we also must learn to shelve many facts and stories gathered about the lives of others when we leave the office. The required—but self-imposed—prohibition against saying too much about our own life provides the necessary environment and time for the patient's narrative to unfold and the therapeutic alliance to develop.

These professional requirements necessitate protective psychological body armor that transfigures like layers of weather-beaten skin over the years and becomes a part of the fabric of our identity, rarely noticed. Yet, as my friend Claire observes, when do we clinicians stop and consider the cost of being the storage vault for other people? Is our capacity to think our own thoughts and creatively transform them recurrently derailed or weakened by being the container of private information that we must shroud?

Even psychotherapists who have been in practice for only a short time have several examples of the requisite artifice. The circumstance can be as simple as running into a patient at a restaurant or in the grocery store with a friend or loved one. A greeting may or may not be exchanged with the patient. You remain silent afterward, but your companion notices the shift in demeanor and asks, "What was that about?" Instinctively, clinicians with more than a few years under the belt screen out public signs of recognition and let the patient take the lead. You may try to divert attention by commenting on the décor around you or resorting to small talk, but your astute companion picks up on your attempted cover: "Oh, this is one of 'those situations' we just don't talk about together, right?"

The secret keeper's quick change in self-state is an expenditure required by the role. One child analyst I know is an experienced clinical social worker who practices in a large metropolitan area. Dawn Higgins has several young patients in her practice whose parents decided to divorce. They go to the same elementary school as her children. One day, Dawn's two sons returned from class with big news about their friends' parents' break-ups. Of course, she already knew these facts but could not say a word. Dawn deflected on the spot and said to the little boys, "Oh my goodness! That's hard news to hear!" Later, she brought her problem to our consultation group for further reflection.

The nodding heads of seven experienced analysts on the Zoom call assured Dawn that each of us had stood in similar shoes ourselves. Our nonverbal, spontaneous reactions were the reassurance that our colleague needed that she wasn't alone. Some laughter and others' sympathetic recollections helped as well.

Dawn knew she had made the right call professionally. Her response was based on all she was taught, all she had subsequently read in clinical literature, and what she had innately incorporated as ethical. But to her mind, her professional role clashed with her values as a mother, and with a principle she was instilling in her boys: to tell the truth. "I put on an act," Dawn said. "Even if one posits that what I did is in the range of telling a so-called white lie, for the good of my patients, I still feel awful. How can I ask my sons not to stretch the truth when I pretended innocence about what I already knew?" Playing her part—the feigned surprise and false affect in front of the boys—temporarily bruised Dawn's sense of herself as a truthful person. While she was assuaged by the group's empathic support, I found myself wondering how these seemingly trivial dilemmas pile up time after time for clinicians.

This is a simple example of a keeper of secrets having a personal, unanticipated impact that benefited from ongoing discussion with trusted colleagues. Given individual personality style and character traits, an issue that stirs up one therapist may not sow seeds of discomfort in another. Yet, it's unlikely that facing fallout from professional cover-ups of one sort or the other can be totally avoided; this observation raises additional questions about the range of predicaments we stumble upon in our role as therapist. It's another reason I believe that being in a profession where keeping secrets is the coin of the realm is not for the faint of heart, mind, or body.

Complicated Ethics

Perhaps because it happens so frequently and subtly in many types of situations in the psychotherapy profession, we tend to deny that a modest degree of deception holds any ramifications whatsoever to our sense of self or our well-being. One can't quibble with Dawn upholding her professional duty to her patients. And, as we have seen, appropriate generational boundaries between children and adults are essential to promote children's capacity to think, reflect, and learn unencumbered by the exigencies of the adult world. Nonetheless, by keeping what she knew to herself, Dawn toggled between her roles as an analyst and a mother, later feeling haunted by shifting demands.

The consultation group supported Dawn by reminding her that an adult's duty to a child is always to protect. We do not disclose what they are too young to absorb or understand. Her incomplete honesty is thus in a protected class of its own (Bonhoeffer, 1965, cited in Bok, 1978) because "the parents' claim on the child is different from the child's claim on the parents. . . 'telling the truth' means something different according to the particular situation in which one stands" (1965/1978, p. 282).

After this self-evident clarification was reexamined, the discussion in the group took a surprising and vexing turn. Momentarily stunned, Dawn replied, "There's no ethical conundrum. That's so obvious now." And then she appended her insight with a spontaneous association. "Something got tangled up in my mind," she reflected. "It's more than juggling conflated roles. Talking it over with the group, I realize that I lost who I was for a minute. At the time, I couldn't think."

Indeed, secret keeping can interfere with the capacity to think clearly, especially when caught off guard or out of context. Therapists know it takes immeasurable mental energy and discretion to keep parcels of information sequestered in their respective vaults. Psychotherapeutic training proffers this ready response when asked about a patient in public: "I can't say anything about that." It may be well intended, but that line certainly didn't fit these circumstances. It rarely does. Saying there is something that you can't say to someone else already lets the cat out of the bag: you know some facts about another individual, and you are not willing to palaver. This morsel invites curiosity and, quite possibly, gossip.

Deception done in the service of others adds up over time. In the group consultation, my colleague sought solace and advice for the conflict she was feeling, along with the vaguely sensed, seamier unconscious ripples of her actions, the absolute force of which one can never be fully aware of in the moment. Dawn asked group members how each of us straddle the different identities we assume in life because of the demands of our various roles—without "losing who we really are." In essence, what are the steps that can be taken to consider what some might categorize as imposture that protect patients? How is work with them protected while not spinning us, the treaters, in a vortex of shame that may simultaneously undermine our personal relationships and the sense of who we are as individuals?

Perhaps you've found yourself in a similar predicament. You have information that you cannot reveal to a friend, loved one, or even another colleague in your community because of your role as therapist. You try to conclude your private conversation or change topics, but your friend or loved one keeps importuning for more information. You become annoyed or angry but are not free to acknowledge that either, lest you give something away. You conclude the talk befuddled, mystified, and unsure about what to do because you could not speak openly about the truths you know.

You might observe some sequelae. You feel an urge to blurt out the private information to dispel internal consternation. Your body tries to siphon off tension by involuntarily twitching, blinking, grimacing, or glancing around. You long, retrospectively, for just the right retort that might throw the curious other off the scent of intimate details you hold, and as you rethink the incident, you spin rejoinders in your mind about how you *should* have shut down the whole unfortunate moment, quietly making a pledge to yourself that you will do better the next time.

If you walked away from the encounter, artfully dodging or without blowing your cover, you may feel assured your professional camouflage remained unscathed and intact. But questions from the rearview mirror linger: What is stirring me up? Did I cross any line in terms of my ethical duties and moral principles? Am I ruminating about what transpired because I'm annoyed or because I couldn't be totally myself and say what was on my mind?

One reason I continue to admire my friend Claire is that she has cultivated so many crafty ways of handling delicate situations over the course of her life, seemingly without fuss. Claire refuses to lie. Her managerial experience helped her to acquire ingenious stratagems to avoid prevarication. She skirts the way she actually feels by emphasizing others' positive qualities or offering a stealth censure.

Like ethicist Sissela Bok, Claire believes that even presumably harmless lies are to be avoided whenever possible because they have the propensity to chip away at both the psyche and the soul. Bok warns that shading the truth, while sometimes inevitable, tends toward doing

> Cumulative harm and expanding deceptive activities. Those who begin with white lies can come to resort to more frequent and more serious ones . . . The aggregate harm from a large number of marginally harmful instances may, therefore, be highly undesirable in the end—for liars, those deceived, and honesty and trust more generally.
>
> (Bok, 1978, p. 60)

Paying attention to the unique, accumulated maneuvers we use to stay mum and to restrain spilling details is an essential first step in fostering essential self-care for professionals whose work requires any degree of concealment.

When Claire asked me to consider the costs of being a therapist, she was implicitly tuning in to more than just the emotional contagion that occurs when carefully listening to and feeling empathy for other peoples' problems. She helped me to perceive the heftier guise a therapist takes on to maintain equanimity in the face of life histories that are anything but "cheerful." Claire exemplifies an ability to contain and transform what she hears, much like a skilled clinician. While I know that intellectual aptitude and emotional intelligence are among her innate gifts, she and I concur that at least part of her dexterity in handling the world is the much practiced, largely unconscious competency required of one who grew up as a person of color in a racially prejudiced society.

As our friendship grew throughout the 1980s and 1990s, the lexicon of privilege and financial disparity in upbringing was rudimentary. We struggled to be straightforward about these differences with each other and were not as direct about them as we are now, a form of unspoken concealment that at the time went largely unaddressed, even among the best of friends. The privations experienced because of race and social class combine with the value Claire places on honesty that spur her to directly tackle uncomfortable subjects in conversation. In contemporary parlance, she faced uncountable microaggressions and "racial enactments" in life since her childhood. Claire subverts the trauma now by staying resolutely calm in rough waters—consider the emotional intelligence cultivated to handle delicate administrative matters with students and to soothe distraught babies—and through offering clever rejoinders without apology.

Taking full measure of the discrepant risks and benefits of camouflage and disguise, Claire observes:

> It's not that I don't see my color, Kassy, as Russ assumed. I've always been aware of the repercussions and got so tired of being 'the first black woman who' whenever I received a promotion or better position. The race issue is unspoken but ever present. I knew long ago that I would need to deal with people as I am. I can't zip off my skin when I walk into a room. You, on the other hand, can pass. When you're asked by people you don't know particularly well what your husband does, are you ever tempted to skirt the truth?

The Therapist's Secret Identities

Therapists unconsciously resort to alter egos while simultaneously ignoring or minimizing their influence. In "Secret Identities in the Lives of Working Clinicians" (2005), David Anderegg urges therapists to "meet" and become friendly with those secret identities. Of the three types he identifies, none connote the noble values and attributes a therapist likes to imagine about oneself.

Martyrdom, desertion, and seduction are descriptors of states of mind the therapist inhabits out of identification with Freud or idealized mentors. These are postures that help us "define ourselves [as] heroic" and are "opportunities to act out archaic fantasies" (p. 333) that ultimately undermine and stultify the patient's and our own growth. Anderegg opines that a culture hostile to the slower, painstaking work of therapy makes the clinician automatically and unconsciously defensive. This plays out repeatedly when we downplay our expertise (martyrdom), abandon psychoanalytic ideas based on circumstance (desertion), or indirectly avoid direct questions about the way we work (seduction) to gain favor with patients and other professionals—attorneys come to mind.

There are "consequences to our not-so-secret identities" (p. 339) that gainsay otherwise solid clinical work and professional self-worth. Careful and ongoing self-assessment of the clinician's secret identities can, according to Anderegg, set the stage for greater openness by the patient to confront the secret identities they keep hidden for fear of stigmatization and shameful reproach.

Implicit in Anderegg's explication is that "secret" and "not-so-secret" identities occur on a continuum that have ethical implications. Several psychodynamic authors have distinguished themselves by candid case reports addressing actual, repressed, or dissociated self-states they noticed inhabiting when with patients. Personal identifiers are not usually disclosed but are part of the therapist's personhood: adoption; prior divorce; remarriage;

adultery; treatment for illness, addiction, or eating disorder; legal problems in the family; financial reversal; religion; and sexual orientation. With the advent of the Internet, telehealth, and web sites, personal facts and areas of specialization are publicized that elicit inquiries from prospective clientele. Consequently, patients know more about the therapist at the outset of treatment and may feel entitled to pose questions that are uncomfortable or that the clinician simply does not want to answer: *Did you choose your specialty because you or a family member struggle with an addiction? Is your expertise in reproductive mental health and infertility gained from personal experience?*

What the therapist wants to keep private may already be known in the practitioner's community, where unscrupulous parties prone to gossip are all too willing to share "confidential information." As I hint throughout the book, this is a self-aggrandizing currency for anyone who shares indiscreetly. It's tempting to gloat about the problems of others, thus narcissistically casting oneself as seer or as above the fray. In the treatment setting, these revelations can create ripples on the conscious-unconscious continuum for both clinician and patient and underlie a stalemate or setback in the treatment.

Some scholars have noticed that anyone can be caught off guard by the extent and degree of their professional camouflage, unaware how it impacts the treatment. A secret identity lay fallow for significant periods of time but eventually bore fruit as the psychic reality of patient and therapist revealed itself in the treatment. What initially seemed like a setback led to opportunities for growth for both parties when the suppressed or dissociated secret identity was no longer sequestered.

Jean Petrucelli, an expert in addictions and a training and supervising psychoanalyst at the William Allen White Institute in New York, has written about a dramatic example of having to lead a double life for the sake of the treatment of a severe bulimic patient. Unbeknownst to her son, the patient's mother called with an urgent request to talk to her. After securing the patient's permission, Petrucelli had a conversation and learned family secrets that the patient was totally unaware of on a conscious level. His father was homosexual; she was now severely ill, had been married twice before, and had also carried on a long-term affair with another man in a distant city while married to her son's father.

This patient's "family was built on secrets and double lives" (Petrucelli, 2010, p. 143), but the therapist understood that the multiple levels of deception were "all in the service of maintaining a surface illusion" (p. 144) that could only be gradually metabolized by her patient. Meanwhile, Petrucelli's professional identity and alliance with her patient were impinged upon because she "became the temporary holder of family secrets and temporarily had to live a double life. I felt my disease in knowing something that I couldn't reveal I knew" (p. 144). She was "the one now trying to talk about what must not be spoken" (p. 146). Only after Petrucelli accepted her role in the enactment could she access her own and her patient's split-off excitement, aggression, and rage—vital elements of each of their identities, where "the real action often is in what is not being seen—the secret" (p. 137).

Alongside striking clinical descriptions of secret identities such as Anderegg's and Petrucelli's are the more common issues and identifiers hinted at earlier in the chapter that concern our common humanity and multiple roles. Until relatively recently, medical issues, marital history, sexual orientation and gender, disabilities, and struggles with one's children have been considered private matters. Insisting on anonymity has been thought to be for the benefit of the treatment. Some clinicians choose not to disclose personal aspects of their life even when that choice disrupts the treatment.

It's understandable. Who wants to be thought of as an unwell person? Just because a patient can read about you on the Internet, do they deserve access to your marital status, sexual orientation, and cultural background? That may still be considered personal information and something you may not want to divulge. But, for example, what complications in the treatment might arise if you don't speak about a noticeable disability? After stinging gossip in your community creates discomfiture that "everybody knows," how do you make space to acknowledge what may be a complex family matter?

Therapists handle these types of boundary considerations between themselves and their patients in different ways, depending on circumstances, but disclosure to patients is less the point than understanding that one is always, to some extent, living with different self-states and circumnavigating private facts that we are conflicted about disclosing. These can morph into a secret identity that takes a toll on the capacity of both parties to think clearly, and the more we are mindful of the influence, the better we tend to ourselves and the patient.

Following a prolonged hiatus to receive treatment for a serious illness, Sandor Abend (1982) returned to practice, visibly impacted by his condition. He decided not to tell most of his patients any personal details of what transpired but encouraged them to elaborate their fantasies. He believed that this approach respected the individual's needs and allowed transference to flourish. But in this post-illness phase, he found himself struggling with a reaction formation: to regain a sense of confidence, efficacy, and self-esteem, he had wanted to return to work too soon. His goal had been to allow full expression of his patients' separation anxiety, his incapacity and possible death, and the anger and abandonment fears. But he found his professional identity at the time strengthened by "holding on to the familiar and far more comfortable role of physician, attentive to and concerned about the anxieties of others, not my own" (p. 372).

While neither the illness nor it having a professional impact was ever in question, Abend discovered that clinicians are prone to keep their guilt, their deeply held gratifications about their occupation, and their impossible ideals to themselves out of fear of "personal exposure of deep, nominally hidden aspects of their own psychological makeup" (p. 378). Urging the need for more study of what information to impart to patients and when, Abend implicitly questions the impact on the clinician's identity of life-altering events and urges exploration of inevitable questions that arise while maintaining strong boundaries and insisting upon personal privacy.

There's no perfect therapeutic stance for ensuring personal privacy in professional relationships, but a particularly strict approach can have a downside that balloons into gaslighting and negatively influences the alliance. This occurs most often when the therapist is bogged down by a sense of conflict, shame, or guilt about their situation. Recently, authorities have championed a stance in which more is gained than lost by taking a welcoming position that encourages the patient to speak to what they suspect, know, or assume about their therapist (Abassi, 2014; A. Pizer, 2016; S. Pizer, 2009).

An unexpected, life-threatening surgery left Stuart Pizer (2009) dealing with a temporary colostomy, which he decided to disclose to his patients. The prolonged aftermath "shifted me to a more right brain mode of being" and self-states of "heightened body experience . . . posttraumatic psychic readjustments . . . management of shame and vulnerability . . . [and] greater absorption of my exposure to near death" (p. 51). He knew, for example, that his colostomy was fetid, and he did not want his patients to deny or dissociate the sensory experience of smelling intestinal gas that he could not control. He chose to urge his patients to be direct about their reactions, even when it meant speaking about the embarrassing odors in the office. Pizer concluded that his newly embodied perceptions modified his capacity to attune to similar splits in his patients that advanced the treatment, but only as he also surmounted subtle shifts in his identity as an analyst—a vulnerable, wounded healer.

Like Stuart Pizer, Ari Pizer (2016) struggled to own his full identity as a blind person with a patient who tried to deny its impact on the therapy. He found that "the negotiation of personal, professional, and disability identities became the crucible for growth, and genuine relatedness" (p. 225). Both accounts address the bidirectionality of the intersubjective space between a therapist and a patient: it is inevitably influenced by the therapist's life circumstances, which the patient may wish to avoid speaking about but can lead to growth when broached in a well-considered manner that sheds light on the patient's dynamics and personal history.

Aisha Abassi questions why little has been written about difficulties in the analyst's private life. Based on her lived experience as mother to a child who transitioned to acknowledge his gender, she did not keep the matter a secret with her family, friends, or professional circle. She knew the fact would eventually reach her patients' ears and that she would address it on an individual basis. In two very different clinical vignettes, Abassi provides details about how this turned out to be the situation and from which vantage she offers her well-honed professional guidance. Patients and therapists must maintain, she says, a capacity to think together in challenging moments:

> I believe things happen in our lives, and that patients may learn about some of them; with others, we may decide to inform patients about ourselves. Our job . . . is to keep working with our patients in the deepest and most honest way we can, and to try to help them understand what information that has been revealed to them by others means to them and what they feel about "knowing" what they now know.
>
> (p. 61)

Indeed, most challenges to the therapist's sense of identity arise from what a patient may already know about the therapist and not disclose. This type of secret keeping is traditionally referenced as a problem that gives rise to countertransference difficulties or overidentifying with the patient. Theodore Jacobs (1987) points out that Joesph Sandler (1976) emphasized how patient and therapist are always influencing each other; it is impossible to remain totally opaque despite protestations of anonymity in the guise of neutrality. Patients always see, and they sense more than they directly acknowledge. These perceptions are often accurate, but the patient requires explicit and repeated permission from the therapist to be open about them. The therapist, on the other hand, has a need, not always conscious, to keep the patient in the dark because personal facts may be embarrassing if exposed. In essence, shame in the countertransference stays secret.

What goes unspoken becomes enacted. Recall from Chapter 2 that Jacobs also described the role of secrets in promoting adolescent separation and individuation (1980, 1987). He elaborates in these papers instances of the analyst's personal loss, professional disappointment, rigid adherence to the frame, or illness. Several patients pieced together observations about him that were not always accurate but were portholes into their psychodynamic issues. Jacobs concludes that a therapist may try to whitewash some small but obvious human frailty by keeping silent in order to avoid a narcissistic wound, guilt, or emotional pain. This cover-up does the treatment no favors when it collides with the patient's own secret-keeping tendencies. Stonewalling also impacts the therapeutic alliance, the development of trust, and transference. Both parties are ultimately left weaker.

Jacobs found that when he heard veiled references to what he had previously wanted to keep private but spoke directly to the patient's fantasies or observations of reality, their memory and other ego functions improved, superego pressures diminished, and their tendencies toward perfectionism and omnipotence could be interpreted. One way of understanding the change is that the patient benefited from identification with the therapist's diminished need to cling to an unconscious secret identity of omniscience or shame. When experienced as more human and reachable in the relationship, the therapist opened a pathway for the patient to be more honest and direct—and hence less clandestine—in the next phase of treatment.

Sometimes, the patient's attack on the clinician's ethical conduct, expertise, and well-being can be quite overt and virulent, leading the therapist to take refuge in defenses such as emotional distancing, boredom, and self-blame. Louise Carignan (1999) treated a bisexual man who recreated his fears in the analysis by disavowing that his analyst was a separate person. He played out his undermining parental relationships via sadomasochistic surrender in the transference that propelled Carignan to become "increasingly (and unduly) preoccupied by my inability to know anything" (p. 916). This patient's misuse of his homosexual and heterosexual partners as "impersonal, interchangeable, dehumanized" objects was concealed for long periods of time and recreated a "collusive relationship with a mother that disavowed his sexuality" (p. 918), which Carignan experienced as a perverse attack on her capacity to think.

Only with ongoing self-analysis of her countertransference could Carignan recover her "autonomy and identity" (p. 920). She had been "manipulated into playing a role" and alternatively "turned into an accomplice [and] voyeur who was tantalized" (p. 924). She concluded that long-standing secrets of significant magnitude, particularly those encased by perverse scenarios, may lead to enactments and intolerable affect that temporarily dislodge the clinician's sense of who she is. These can ultimately be worked through as the patient is able "to consolidate his sense of identity" (p. 925) and repair his internal object world, where separation and individuation occur, and truthfulness prevails.

The potential for ethical transgression, destructive secret keeping, and challenges to the therapist's identity as healer congeal in Sue Grand's detailed case report of a professionally successful but contemptuous patient who could not separate from her symbiotic mother (Grand, 2003). The analyst, still early in her career at the time, found herself unable to establish a secure frame with her sadistic and voracious patient, whose demands for extra therapeutic contact and maternal succor, escalation of somatic symptoms, and hatred hid how the treatment was helping her. The patient started dating for the first time, but she complained that analysis was making her and her mother physically sick. The analyst knew the patient lied, and, correspondingly, she felt she had lied to her patient by virtue of her inability to address her own countertransference shame, guilt, and hate in a therapeutic manner.

Grand's patient was eventually able to terminate the analysis, marry, and have a child, but not before Grand believed she committed ethical errors when she lost capacity for introspection that precipitated multiple enactments. She asserts that collective silence about quagmires of this kind is common but destructive to the psychotherapy profession because the clinician "is in possession of a secret that must be discovered but cannot be revealed" (p. 491) for substantial periods of time. This scenario imposes on the analyst a false identity of one who does not make mistakes and is neither supposed to "speak nor write of our failures and destructive interventions" (p. 493) that inevitably arise in challenging situations.

Carignan and Grand discovered one secret identity that clinicians are prone to wear when treating severe characterological disturbance: the mask of omniscience. This costume is a malignant variant of the more benign, everyday professional camouflage. It is particularly hard to detect in the throes of the tumult created by primitively organized or destructive patients who divest themselves of noxious and aggrandizing internal objects via projection, stirring mayhem within the therapist who only retrospectively grasps the concomitant impingement on one's personhood and value system.

Both types of masquerades, as we have seen, have the potential to derail the capacity to think clearly about oneself and the other person. Fortunately, they can, to some extent, be ameliorated by the self-righting processes we take up next, which are enlivening staples of therapeutic nourishment.

Containment and Transformation

Holding, containing, and transforming all the information a therapist takes in on a given day are part of an acquired skill set that grows over the years of practice.[1] These abilities—sometimes weighty and emotionally taxing, but informative—become an essential requirement when we hear secrets.

What is shared by a patient may be an affront to our personal values. Some comments may puncture our confidence. We are still required to stay nonjudgmental—and yet fully engaged—regarding the content of what we take in. Muffling an audible gasp, knowing when to raise an eyebrow to emphasize a point, remaining stone-faced, and coping with an entire range of physical signals—from yawning to nausea—are skills we have built. They are responses to what we our hearing—our body's way of telling us that the patient's story is influencing our emotional container. All the while, we try to sense what the patient is trying to convey that isn't fully verbalized—or what they may not want us to know, such as deep psychic wounds that exude as yet unspeakable pain, terror, and abandonment.

At such moments, the task of the clinician is to step back and pose a question far easier to ask oneself than to directly answer: What am I being asked to hold? The answer is whatever is emanating from the patient that cannot yet be fully known or understood. And are the conditions in the environment experienced as safe? Can we begin to think together to begin the transformational process of finding words that promote healthier defenses and greater accessibility to prior impingements on their mind and body? Do we need more time to simply be together and speak about seeming trivialities and the day-to-day? Would that create the conditions for trust to evolve naturally? As my colleague Robert Galatzer-Levy pointed out in a discussion group of senior analysts, "When it appears that you are doing 'nothing' you are always doing something in the treatment" (personal communication, 2018; see also Gabbard, 1989).

Theoretically derived from the earliest relationship with a primary caretaker who tolerated pain, metabolized it for the infant, and offered it back in manageable bits, the capacity to contain later enables a child to process thoughts on their own. From there, the individual mind grows (Bion, 1962, 1975; Borgogno, 2022; Brown, 2012). Intersubjectivity flourishes as the baby reintrojects what the caregiver has transformed, especially "very painful feelings of need" (Reiner, 2012, p. 15). Thus, expression of one's own thoughts is an inherently relational process that promotes coherence and integration of the true self essential for living a vibrant life (Borgogno, 2022; Brown, 2012; Grotstein, 2000, 2007; Little, 1981, 1990; Reiner, 2012, 2017). Sadly, the seemingly paradoxical processes that "facilitate a sense of oneness beyond boundaries of each individual self (and) simultaneous awareness of separateness and at-one-ment with the other" (Reiner, 2012, pp. 18–19) are, to some extent, lacking in our patient-to-be.

Psychoanalyst Margaret I. Little speaks to the capacity to contain another person's angst by revealing details of her personal analysis with D. W. Winnicott (Little, 1990). After two previous psychotherapeutic treatments that proved somewhat beneficial, Little turned to Winnicott for additional help. She was terrified by unremitting depression, had difficulty enjoying sex, and felt blocked in her pursuit to become a psychoanalyst.

Winnicott provided a holding environment for Little that included his actual office setting of "physical comfort, warmth, quiet, and absence of interruption," along with an "attitude of acceptance, encouragement, and response" (Little, 1990, p. 89). His observations about the difficulties she had in speaking her truth combined with reciprocity of candor and humanity in the dyad that conveyed safety and hopefulness. Over time, Little revealed details of early deprivation (i.e., split-off and repressed memories of her developmental history), where she felt annihilated and "an appendage" of her disturbed mother and emotionally aloof father.

These unearthed facts, which were blocking her true self, emerged in the treatment, which made Little deeply regressed and furious at Winnicott. She later concluded that his patience and endurance of her emotional explosions was key to recovery. In addition to environmental provision of a secure base, Little says he sometimes metaphorically "held" her with his wit, playfulness, and sincerity in answering her direct questions. He did not rush in with interpretations. When he made one, it had profound impact.

To illustrate the breakdown in an individual's capacity to think and the ethical challenges that can arise from it, we take one relevant clinical example and one example from memoir. These also demonstrate what can occur when information is compartmentalized and therefore goes unbroached between individuals who seek forthrightness and depth. Members of any dyad cannot join together in a mutual, and ultimately life-affirming, process of giving back and forth when important thoughts and feelings are withheld or fabricated. Intersubjective space collapses, distorting the normal shape of human subjectivity. A relational process based on owning and sharing one's truth is precisely what allows for mental transformation and growth over the life cycle.

Adolescents and adults have ongoing needs for emotional recognition and support; the use of language is an essential feature of those sustained bonds. Open discourse transforms emotions and diminishes coercion. In essence, creative capacities are undermined without the mutative processes of holding and containment that enable facing one's truth, however painful, and negotiating the forward arc required for authentic engagement.

The Safe-Deposit Box

Rebecca Samuels, a thirty-nine-year-old hospital chaplain and married mother of two, called in crisis.

> My need is urgent. My problem is irresolvable and existential. I've never been in therapy and don't want it now, but this isn't something I'm kicking upstairs to senior clergy. Can you see me immediately? I don't think it will take long to figure out an answer.

I was puzzled by the message but had time in my calendar for what I assumed would be a short-term consultation for someone in the helping profession who seemed in peril. I planned to meet with Rebecca a few times and make recommendations, perhaps for further psychotherapy or analysis.

In our first meeting, Rebecca told me it would take several individual sessions for her to feel "comfortable enough to put my issue front and center," but, in the meantime, she needed medicine immediately. Anxious, sleepless, and continually preoccupied, she worried she might be losing her grip on reality. By all appearances, her life was completely normal, but Rebecca realized she was flagging at home and at work. "This isn't like me at all," she said, "I like comforting others—patients, and staff alike. I'm not able to show up for anybody these days—not even my husband and kids."

Although Rebecca's distress was disquieting for both of us, I sensed that in this situation it was not in her interest to rush to relieve anxiety with medication. I sided with her resistance to not reveal the difficulty immediately and to face her dilemma only when she felt she was ready. I said, "Words will come. Let the disturbance reside between us and see what emerges. Try to remember the gist of Pascal's aphorism: *All of humanity's problems stem from man's inability to sit quietly.*"

Meanwhile, doing so was torturous for both of us. When Rebecca came to my office, she exuded foreboding that she projected into me. I understood my task as temporarily holding this maelstrom of affect and subterranean storyline despite feeling impatient, confused, and apprehensive. Why was I nearly gasping for breath when her session was over? How long would it take her to get to her point? By alluding to the importance of the space between us where the disturbance could eventually be understood and processed, I was speaking to my belief in the transformational power of holding and containment that enable thought to emerge.

Rebecca's story leaked out over a couple of weeks. She had apparently run into Joe, a public defender for the mentally ill, in the hospital cafeteria where she worked part-time. They hadn't seen each other in years but had had a serious romantic relationship when she was in seminary and he in law school. Rebecca had fallen deeply in love with Joe and was heartbroken when he suddenly broke off their romance, ostensibly because he was an atheist.

Rebecca didn't need to tell me she still carried the torch for Joe despite her professed love for her spouse Dan. When Joe asked her for coffee to catch up on their lives, she found herself primping as if she were going out on a date. She saw no need to tell her husband about the meeting even though he was aware of the prior relationship. This is how she rationalized her decision: "I would never have an affair with Joe and wreck my wonderful family."

Joe and Rebecca continued to get together for lunch or "just to talk" a couple of times a week despite my warning that she was playing with fire. The clandestine meetings had, in fact, created a secret in her marriage that was potentially destructive. When she began to argue with me, I tried to put my somatic countertransference reactions to use and suggested that I thought she was conflicted between her resurfaced excitement about Joe and the shame and dread of discovery after their reconnection. Her anxiety and sexual arousal left her breathless. Her feelings were the upstream instigators of the symptoms she complained about in our first appointments.

The get-togethers continued in public as Rebecca remained in weekly psychotherapy to simmer and to try to sort through her feelings. I silently formulated my role as a temporary repository for her secret liaison and the amalgam of feelings she would need to process through, over time, to be able to move head. Something was amiss, however, and I couldn't put my finger on it. In our sessions, I found myself uncharacteristically unable to think clearly and suspected that I was caught up in collusion with Rebecca.

Then a proposal took her predicament to a new level. Rebecca called for an extra session. Overwhelmed but contrite, she pleaded, "Please tell me what to do about this situation. I have no idea. I can't think. I've lost my mind."

She tearfully related the backstory. Joe asked to meet in Rebecca's private office. She agreed, despite her better judgment. There he presented a tiny box. She stared at the diamond ring set in platinum and surrounded by sapphires. "Joe knelt on one knee," she told me. He said to her,

> I just want you to know one thing. Then I am leaving for good. It has always been you. I know you can't—you won't—and I really don't want you to leave Dan. You'll ruin your life. But this ring is yours with all my love.

Joe then stood up, turned, and dashed out of the room and slammed the door shut behind him, leaving Rebecca to gaze at the jewels, stunned.

The big secret—what had been behind the curtain of our therapeutic relationship so far—slipped through her lips. Rebecca told me that her original call to my office weeks before was prompted by this veiled marriage proposal and the heartbreak she could not withstand carrying on her own. I suddenly knew why my body reacted anxiously in the initial sessions and why I felt dazed, almost crestfallen, about what to do after Rebecca left. Nothing I said seemed to have been helpful. I realized that I had been meeting with Rebecca under a ruse all this time and offering her a point of view that she could not make use of because the clandestine get-togethers and eventual admission of love occurred *before she came to my office the first time.* Only now did she trust our work enough to allow herself to be flooded with anguish and despair about her feelings for Joe and to tell the truth.

Like an adolescent seeking solace from a potentially disappointed or angry parent, Rebecca implored,

> Please try to understand. Don't get mad at me. I could not break Joe's or Dan's heart. I can't keep the ring at home. It's a ticking bomb. I can't give it up either. There's no solution. Tell me what I should do.

I knew it would take substantially more time for Rebecca to sort through her dilemma to have any substantive psychological impact. I also recognized that she was pleading with me to keep her secret contained in our relationship, where it could be openly spoken about and processed with time. How could both be accomplished with minimal damage, giving all parties sufficient space to gain perspective? I suggested to Rebecca that we needed time to understand the complexities of the situation that beset her and process through them.

Rebecca returned to the next session, pleased. After we last met, she had had a moment of inspiration. She had gone directly to her bank and secured a safe-deposit box to store the ring. Only she had access to the box. She could bide time until she knew what to do next. If she felt moved to "visit" the ring for private reasons and to consider her options, she told me she could do so.

I reminded my patient that this safe-deposit box would put pressure on her to keep her story private, to avoid personal and professional exposure. This might be more difficult to do than it seemed: there is a human compulsion to make a confession to more than one person, particularly with issues of the heart (Gross, 1951; Margolis, 1966, 1974). Renting the secret box to store her secret ring had actually created another secret. I wondered whether something from her past or family history was repeating by this secret within a secret. The theme was even being played out in our relationship, and it would require incremental reconstruction of her history.

Consciously stowing her ring and the secrets it held in a safe place was simultaneously a concrete symbol for the psychodynamic concept of holding. Silently, I hypothesized that the therapeutic process would serve as a necessary container in which Rebecca could metabolize complex feelings based on personal history that she would gradually "take back into herself" to help her make a pivotal life decision. No harm was done by waiting, contemplating, and arriving at a well-considered decision.

This perspective contradicted the advice given to me years before by esteemed family therapy instructors at the Menninger Clinic. When treating individuals or couples experiencing an emotional or actual affair, these mentors advised, "one must make a choice." When an adult loves two people simultaneously, it is the therapist's duty to facilitate that decision by confronting the secret keeper about the harm they are doing to the three adults involved and to the other key victims, usually children. While I will never be precisely sure what these teachers would say if faced with the same set of circumstances, I can imagine they would intuit the compromise formation the patient and I were enacting and suggest that I be clear: Rebecca should either send the ring back to Joe or immediately tell Dan what had happened.

My own sense was that Rebecca would leave treatment before budging, so the training ideal was moot. She deceived me from the beginning and was obviously terrified of reprisal. I made the clinical judgment to hold onto the new information about the ring and its whereabouts with her, for as long as needed, to clarify the threads that confounded her. Provision of a confidential setting seemed essential to help Rebecca gain insight and minimize fallout that likely would reverberate for the rest of her life. Establishing trust and a sense of safety could not be taken for granted in this situation, but they were indispensable first steps (Allen, 2022; Brockman, 2023; Peebles, 2022).

It didn't turn out the way I envisioned. Rebecca continued psychotherapy for another three months, and then quit. While we processed areas of her life that touched on her feelings for Joe and Dan, she made no decisions. Then Rebecca mysteriously dropped off the map, despite my efforts to contact her.

To the best of my knowledge, the ring remained in the safe-deposit box throughout our work. For all I know, it is still there. It's an unsatisfying conclusion, but one familiar to many experienced clinicians. As much as we hope that dialogue fosters mental growth and shared communication in which secrets can be released, sometimes the therapist never learns the outcome. We are left holding the bag—or the symbolic ring, as the case may be.

Just as Jean Petrucelli, Louise Carrigan, and Sue Grand showed in their clinical examples, I found myself temporarily playing a role and inhabiting a false identity imposed by my dysregulated patient. While I believed in the moment that the only intervention I could make was to slow things down and follow Rebecca's lead, I wish, in retrospect, that I had interpreted the bind she placed us both in.

Hindsight leads me to consider what might have happened if I had been more cognizant of how my identity had been co-opted. I might have said something as simple as

> You know, your secrets are putting us both in a predicament. Joe left you with a mess by giving you the ring, and I think you are doing a similar thing with me. You're having trouble seeing that Joe was aggressively asking you to hold something for him too. That is not an act of 'forever,

ideal love.' I find myself wondering whether the space of therapy is the 'safe-deposit box' for your anger and disappointment toward Joe that is easier to dump here rather than to close out. I also think you're angry with me for pointing out the layers of secrets you created for yourself that are strangulating your ability to act in your own interests.

I suspect that Rebecca sought out therapy to find a reservoir to hold her feelings in a state of suspended animation indefinitely. Perhaps the secret instigated an attack on the process of thinking itself. The mental and inter-personal paralysis created by this type of ongoing concealment leads to breakdown of knowledge formation and a distortion in communication, what Wilfred Bion called "K" (see Chapter 5; Bion, 1970,1975; Brown, 2012; Grotstein, 2007; Orgad, 2014).

Stunning examples on the impingement of thought and ethical decision-making kindled from extraordinary secret keeping are ever pre-sent in our consultation rooms and professional literature but extend well beyond psychotherapeutic practice. Novels, short stories, biographies, and autobiographies are rife with similar truths. We now turn to another data source to elucidate the ramifications—the contemporary memoir of Lucinda Franks.

Secret Wars in the Mind

In 2007, investigative journalist Lucinda Franks published *My Father's Secret War: A Memoir* that described her father's role as an espionage agent in Europe during World War II and, afterward, stateside in the early years of the Cold War. This debonair, polished businessman, husband, and father of two daughters tried to keep this secret life totally sealed off from his family. Franks's memoir recounts how she discovered much about the life of her father, Tom, as he physically deteriorated in his sixties and even-tually succumbed to dementia.

Only after years of going on a fact-finding mission—sorting through boxes of stored memorabilia, making discreet inquiries to his military friends and business associates, and picking up clues from interviews he agreed to give to the Museum of Jewish History's Holocaust Memorial in New York—did she learn the astounding details that had influenced her development and early adult life. Tom Franks's eyewitness account gave historical documentation of the liberation from Nazi concentration camps where genocide had occurred. Listening to the horrific details in his recordings let Lucinda appreciate, and to some extent later forgive, the inscrutable and seemingly aloof father who repeatedly bore witness to the sight and smell of corpses and death, disease and starvation, and anguished survivors of body injuries, psychological torture, and family loss.

Her father's military oath of silence came with significant costs. Reminiscent of the promise my patient Landon made on his mother's behalf (Chapter 2), Frank's memoir is filled with poignant and insightful speculations about the high price paid, viewed from the perspective of a family member. When one takes on a role where maintaining confidential information for a lifetime is a requirement, where is the tipping point for hearing or knowing too much? Does witnessing the horrific or engaging in deceptive actions make some individuals susceptible and not others? What mechanisms can be used to soothe the self or briefly stop ruminations, but leave loved ones shut out, lonely, and yearning for interpersonal contact and intimate connection?

Stargazing, shooting firearms, and collecting insects became Tom Franks's defenses. His daughter speculates that by middle age, her father employed his hobbies to serve as essential psychological glue. On the surface, he functioned at a high level, but to do so he required help; he was mentally harboring so much pain. As she meticulously pulls together details of the clandestine work and the mortifying ethical decision points involved in espionage duties, the author gains perspective and respect for her father' multifold ability to cover his tracks—all the while losing track of the man he was and aspired to be.

The author's detective work about her father continued over years. She undertook it because she ached to understand the man she once adored but came to despise because of his remote affect, enigmatic behaviors, alcoholism, and infidelity. Her father never spoke to his family about his heroic espionage duties. He also posed as an SS officer at Buchenwald and other concentration camps to assist Allied forces strategizing the initial liberation efforts of Holocaust survivors. Like many secret keepers, he left clues behind in files and boxes. When Franks made her first discoveries, she tried to ask her father questions about some facts she had pieced together. He still refused to talk.

Franks's efforts eventually led the memoirist to seek out her father's mistress, a woman he had loved for many years and whom Franks initially loathed. She assumed the woman was responsible for her parents' breakup. Daughter and mistress slowly established a bond of friendship; Franks corroborated and synthesized what she had pulled together about her father and, most importantly, how much he did, in fact, love his family. Tom Franks indeed was, according to his mistress, disturbed about the ethics of his ongoing espionage duties after the war in the 1950s. His mistress confided how overwhelming and destructive the choices were for the man she also loved, but he could not stop punishing himself for deeds he was ordered to do:deeds that he believed were morally corrupt. Attempting to explain the layers of duplicity, trauma, and silence required by his espionage assignments, his mistress described her own version of the price he paid:

I wanted him to talk more about it, but he wouldn't. You know, generally I succeeded in getting beneath that crust he has. After the war, I would question him until he told me what was on his mind. *He had to talk, I knew that, or he was going to explode inside.*

(p. 110, italics added)

Once again, a witness of someone who loved a person with a secret life tells us that there is an essential need to find a safe place where truths can be let out of the vault. Tom Franks's decision to not reveal himself was a complex ethical compromise undertaken for everyone's best interest at the time but ultimately disruptive to family members' stability, their sense of reality, and, presumably, at times, his own. His affective burden was apparent but unarticulated in the household. Orgad (2014) explains that family secret keeping to such a complex degree as Tom Franks's is "corrosive" and not "communicative." Individuals are prevented from knowing each other, "rendering truth inaccessible, un-nameable, and un-usable . . . a joint unconscious attack on a family's truth-generating space" (p. 95).

In her journey, Lucinda Franks found others who verified her suppositions; their conversations and her project helped her process previously unknown and unprocessed mental experience, creating the necessary container in which she could access precious facts, think her own thoughts, and make emotional links to her father. While clinicians are rarely exposed to this degree of concealment in the consultation room, some of our patients come from backgrounds where extraordinary truths have been sequestered for decades. We learn from Franks's memoir that the capacity for reflective function and owned subjectivity can be compromised to the detriment of mental and physical health. Like others, she couldn't untangle many facts until after her loved one's death. Her research and discussion with interviewees provided the holding space—other minds—and containment she required to mourn and, to some extent, heal the wounds left after years of failed communication and stunted intimacy between herself and her father.

Conclusion

The therapeutic process that involves listening to and keeping the secrets of patients raises ethical challenges that are different for every clinician. The scope of these concerns is broad. Whether knowingly or unwittingly, therapists adopt a range of strategies that safeguard the revelation of entrusted private information. At the same time, they must be attuned to the myriad ways these secrets impact others in their lives.

Ethical decision-making is facilitated by a greater awareness of attributes the clinician takes on in the work: it may be as simple as the day-to-day donning of a "protective camouflage" or it may involve inhabiting longer-term but subtle shifts in self-states. The evolution of professional identity and how it can be inadvertently or temporarily shaped by the secrets we hold for patients is an elusive force. We can try to remain aware of it, but the shifts can also take the clinician by surprise. Each new topic in therapy may raise questions for which there are rarely hard-and-fast answers. Openly acknowledging the presence and influence of these challenges and learning how therapists in similar circumstances deal with them promote reflection. None of us is alone in this.

Expanded awareness of unnoticed and unspoken ways therapists conceal aspects of ourselves to facilitate treatment helps us remain steadfast in the work and ethically in line with our professional values. These challenges interfere with the process of reflective thought. Clinical examples and even memoirs like Lucinda Franks's can serve as cautionary tales about the importance of maintaining the capacity to think clearly in the heat of unexpected revelations that evoke strong responses in the treater. If the therapist stays vigilant about ongoing ethical decision points and potential side effects brought about by the work, it *is* possible to remain open, thoughtful, and creative—even when serving as the storage vault of particularly disturbing information.

Note

1 I employ the terms "holding" and "containing" interchangeably as clinical shorthand for the mental and psychological functions the therapist takes on, similar to what Little (1981, 1987) found Winnicott did for her and what she later strove to provide for her patients. This general usage continues in the field, particularly in teaching and supervision, although the concepts have continued to evolve and, in some quarters, take on highly specific and nuanced meaning (see Auchincloss & Samberg, 2012). For that reason, holding is a foundational concept of D. W. Winnicott and his followers in the British Middle School, whereas the rubric of container, or contained, emanates from the discoveries of W. R. Bion (1962, 1970). Despite important technical differences in application in contemporary psychodynamic practice, both converge to encompass the requirement of the primary caretaker to emotionally contact with the infant's primitive, chaotic mental world and provide soothing and understanding. In essence, one thinks the thoughts for the child, so the child is able to eventually think for himself (Bion, 1975), but only after he is sensually "held" and soothed (Winnicott); from these anlagen the pliable and essential intersubjective space necessary for growth and relationships emanates. When there is a deficit in these earliest caretaker provisions, the capacity for physical self-care, let alone formation of thought, breaks down; requirements necessary for self-development (e.g., sleep, solitude, play, thinking, dreaming, creativity) also wither. For parsing of the technical, clinical, and theoretical differences between Winnicott's "holding" and Bion's "container/contained," see Symington and Symington (1996); Grotstein (1997, 2007); Ogden (2004a, b, 2007); Reiner (2012, 2017), who provide essential expansions, comparisons, and referents.

7   Hidden Talents and Abilities

Professor Alejandra Castillo had nothing to hide. She was confident in her expertise and forthright in her opinions.

As she weaved her way through the portico leading to the Department of Romance Languages, her eyes rolled upward again to the ugly gray ceiling. A seat of learning is a sacred place. Why had the college administrators been so careless when choosing the architectural firm to make necessary repairs? She felt a tug to stop, immediately change course, and allow her paisley heels to lead her to the college administration offices, where she would speak her mind.

Her reflections reverberated late Friday after her last analytic session of the week. Professor Castillo was annoyed. The feeling behind her criticism of the university's carelessness opened the gateway for a rush of associations when she returned to my office Tuesday. She was letting us both know how far she had come in her treatment. It was easier for her to claim her voice and openly acknowledge conflict and anger. Now, instead of side-stepping her reactions, she reflected on them and owned them. Sometimes, she even got a kick out of challenging authority.

Everyone in her department privately agreed that the open-air gallery would have been gorgeous and historically accurate had the designers selected the terra-cotta color palette Professor Castillo recommended. She had served as the college's volunteer advisor to the architecture company. Her eagle eyes easily detected nuances in shades of soothing green that she favored for the classroom. The firm's somber selection of grays smothered the finely textured Spanish walls, casting a subliminal pall.

In the classroom, Professor Castillo sought every means she could to convey to her students the vitality, warmth, and sensuality of the diverse cultures that inhabited her native Iberian Peninsula. As she quietly prepared to teach her seminars, she experienced a familiar frustration with hierarchies that she would turn against herself, self-sabotaging with writing block and delayed reports. Today, she decided to make positive use of her self-observation, reverse course, and offer some hard-won advice to her

DOI: 10.4324/9781003471578-8

students. She quoted her favorite Cervantes maxims to the advanced class in Spanish literature: "Be slow of tongue and quick of eye." "Believe there are no limits but the sky."

By this time in her analysis, she and I were well versed in some of these less-conscious motives that propelled the professor to infuse undergraduates with intellectual enrichment that would nourish them for a lifetime. Another motive for teaching was generativity—bestowing to her students the encouragement and direction that she wished she had received more of in young adulthood. As she put it, "I want each one to get good advice and opportunities that I didn't know existed when I was a student."

Linguistically and artistically gifted, Professor Castillo reveled in exploring language, reading widely, and working with her hands to make fine textiles. The favorite part of her daily teaching round was an individual tutorial with a struggling student. Still, she couldn't wait to drive home, enjoy her husband's increasing mastery of Castilian asados, and still have time to draw or weave on her Schacht Wolf Pup loom.

When I, her psychoanalyst, moved my professional office from the medical school to a private space downtown, I was certain she noticed that I picked up a few of her decorating tips over the years of our association. The professor was the kind of woman too polite to mention the contrast colors, knotted wool rug, and wing wall. She let out a hearty laugh of mutual recognition only after I made a point of bringing these facts into our conversation, a necessary prompt for her to own what she saw, who she was, and how much she perceived within the intersubjective spaces that constitute human relatedness.

More than once, we crafted strategies for turning down colleagues who urged her to take on the role of department chair or apply for the position of associate dean. Professor Castillo knew they meant well and admired her. She hated to say no. In treatment, we worked hard to help her cultivate what I term "a healthy sense of ruthlessness" in order to protect time and space for herself that she initially experienced as withholding. I reminded her that time is a commodity one can easily surrender to others and later regret.

In fact, Professor Castillo entered treatment in early midlife to disentangle herself from a web of personal priorities that she relinquished early on. She grieved the suppression of her fascination with architectural design. She spoke to the nurturer role she played in her family of origin. Gradually, she acknowledged the weariness and resentment that arose when she gave too much of herself away to others. She saw how this played out time and time again in her adolescent and later adult friendships. As she neared the end of her analysis, Professor Castillo reviewed with me this web of choices and disappointments and set an ending date for five months hence.

As I frequently pointed out to her, one does not mourn only the people lost to death: we also mourn all the potential lives we could have had in order to fully invest in the life we do have. Developing a resilient self is a lifelong project that requires ongoing psychological maintenance, is never fully completed, and sometimes feels like a violent act of self-sacrifice when bidding farewell to who one might have been or what one could have accomplished.

"I think I know just what you mean today as I lie here on your analytic couch," she said.

> I'm recalling my first day in geometry class in tenth grade. The books were handed out. I paged through mine quickly. It all made sense to me—immediately and intuitively. I looked at the diagrams and skipped ahead to the trigonometry sections. Cosine and sine—the teacher didn't have to say a word. I *saw* it.

The story popped out of nowhere. She hadn't been keeping a conscious secret. I was surprised. Professor Castillo appeared to take it in her stride, like she always knew this part of her history. But an important detail had spontaneously bubbled up from the underbrush. Could it be possible that both of us had disavowed this highly specific aspect of her abilities? What was going on between us and being enacted that needed to be further understood?[1]

She continued her mathematical musing.

> Practical trigonometry is still great fun. I can walk into a room, see the angles, how everything fits together. You know how I love to chat up construction guys that I meet on projects and offer an idea or two. But I haven't thought of that first geometry class for years.

Rubbing her solar plexus, she said,

> I notice it right here. The room is swirling now. I feel seasick. My life could have turned out so differently. Maybe I could have been, *really should have been*, an architect. How many years have we been talking around this subject in my treatment?

I was glad she couldn't see me plop back in my chair as if pushed off a bungee-jump platform. Geometry pleasurable? Really? Who thinks this way? "A line is the shortest distance between two points" is all that was ever easy for me to assimilate on the subject. The point now was, however, that Professor Castillo just added another strand to her autobiography, another line of inquiry for us to pursue. I had to recover my bearings to stay with her in the moment.

The talent for geometry was implied, of course, in her penchant for all things design related, but up to this moment, the fact of it as an inherent ability from childhood was never explicitly stated in just this way. For her, the reminiscence offered pleasure and piquancy; had all the pieces been put into place and nurtured years before, her life trajectory might have been different. This added layer of loss was something for us to look at squarely, take stock of, and place into the simmering "pot of letting go" before she fully let go of the analysis.

For me the lesson had a different, humbling vertex. How often do we miss abilities of those we think we know well? Was it possible that Professor Castillo and I had colluded to disavow aspects of this particular gift? If so, why did it become accessible at this moment? What transpires between caregivers of all kinds—parents and grandparents, teachers, and those of us in the helping professions—to miss an aptitude that was in plain sight the whole time? Talent, ambition, ability—these are the kinds of secrets that are prone to remain silent until coaxed to the surface and given space to be voiced, not only to a listener but also to oneself.

Discovering Inner Treasures

Unearthing an unknown talent or ability occurs relatively frequently in psychodynamic psychotherapy and psychoanalysis. The meaning of the word "secret" includes that which is concealed, set apart, and needing protections (Chapter 1), and indeed, individuals often stow away their hidden treasure inside the psyche when they perceive that it might harm essential attachment relationships. Unconscious dynamics can make secret abilities seem to vanish, but psychotherapy, and other kinds of caring relationships, may help recover them.

Human potential contracts when it is not recognized and nurtured. Without sufficient positive feedback from within the family, school, or cultural environment, ability goes underground—that is, becomes repressed, sequestered, or dies off, especially when it is perceived as damaging, dangerous, or odd. But remove some of the roadblocks to seeing and appreciating a talent and watch aptitudes begin to take form. Tendrils of new growth quickly sprout. Hidden treasures begin to flourish when a truly involved, interested person carefully listens and bears witness. It seems almost magical.

Winnicott's aphorism that "it's a joy to be hidden but a disaster not to be found" (1963, p. 185) captures just this point. Here, Winnicott is underscoring the indispensable requirement for individuals to cultivate competency when a caregiver provides sufficient private space to discover and learn. At the same time, that caregiver must sense when it is the right time to perk up and show that they are paying attention. The delighted smile or praise of a parent captures this enlivened unfolding for the child. In the process of being seen by another person, we are found.

When natural endowment and innate skills are ignored or even quashed, capabilities languish. One surprising finding of the long-term Menninger Psychotherapy Project (Appelbaum, 1977, 1978, 1981; Kernberg, Burstein, Coyne, Appelbaum, et al., 1972; Wallerstein, 1986, 1992) was that a bevy of newfound capabilities blossomed in adult psychiatric inpatients and outpatients (as measured by an extensive array of projective and intelligence tests) within just two years of receiving intensive psychotherapy or psychoanalysis. An expressive approach that focused on the therapist-patient relationship had a high level of impact on even the most severe characterological problems, borderline personality disorder included. Both supportive and expressive psychological treatments were discovered to enhance ego strength, increase motivation, and diminish externalization onto the environment as a source of one's problems. Given those conditions, individuals matured.[2]

For these and other reasons, I'm always on the lookout for patients' hidden gifts and latent abilities and was profoundly perplexed by missing this one for years. Professor Castillo defended against full recognition of her talent because it is painful to stare down the paths of what might have been. Confronting these what-ifs can be a mortifying experience because it means taking full responsibility for living one's life in the present while discerning the interdigitation between imperfect environmental provisions and one's bad internal objects. Had any of these forces been a little different, the way might have been smoothed for different choices. My failure to pick up on Professor Castillo's latent cues derived from a quantum of envy I harbored for gifts she had that I did not. My grounded feet prevented a near catapult from the Stressless rocker and I shook my head in dismay. The rueful moment of truth rekindled a personal—and embarrassing—memory.

Remember to Ask

At the beginning of my career, a group of staff and students at the Menninger Clinic worked together on the diagnostic workup and initial, evolving treatment plan for a highly distraught but charming young inpatient. We assembled at the formal case conference, routinely set at four weeks into a patient's stay. Next steps in treatment were ferreted out then. The team members believed we had done a fine job of pulling together pertinent facts, getting a well-rounded picture of Ms. Greenwood's individual and family issues, and forming a rudimentary therapeutic alliance. It was one of my first experiences of intense interdisciplinary teamwork.

The patient's presentation was unusual, but the psychiatrist team leader was sure of the way forward. He had even begun to draft a short paper about the case. We thought we knew our patient well. We had worked with

Ms. Greenwood for an entire month! We didn't think we needed much help from the esteemed senior clinician assigned to review the workup and offer constructive advice about the treatment plan. Wasn't it a waste of time to get another opinion when everything was moving along quite nicely?

I'm now sure that the *éminence grise* sensed our smugness from the start. Team members gave their discipline's unique perspective, conclusions were synthesized, and the consensus pointed to the route forward. The consultant waited until near the end of the meeting. Everything seemed to be on course and wrapping up when he stopped us in our tracks.[3]

He said,

> Yes, I agree. It does seem to be proceeding well so far for Ms. Greenwood in the 'holding environment' of the hospital. I have just one more question to ask the team members. Who can tell me this patient's 'secret talent'?

Papers stopped shuffling. Heads turned to face the venerable teacher. Surely one of us knew or would hazard a guess. Stymied, there was total silence. No one wanted to humiliate themselves. No one knew.

He paused. Having gotten our attention, he then took his lesson a step further.

"Let me give you a hint," he quipped. "It's an unusual hobby for a young woman to have. And she's so good at it."

Now we were quite uncomfortable. The feminists among us had our hubris plucked. Finally, as if releasing a gold doubloon from his fingertips, he leaned back, faced the team, and opened his hands.

"Chess!" he exclaimed. "She plays chess."

Having snared our attention, the consultant proffered another educational nugget.

He said, "Always remember to ask patients about their talents and interests. They don't tell us unless they know we want to know."

Thus, the therapist must be receptive to buds of creativity and productivity while paradoxically maintaining space for these capacities to take firmer root. When the patient is impinged upon or ignored, their maturational strivings go unnoticed and unwelcomed, and the ineluctable drive to separate is thwarted (Eagle, 2018; Khan, 1974, 1983).

It's a lesson Dr. Karl Menninger underscored throughout his teaching that stands the test of time and will rarely let you down. I recall how he would stride into our didactic seminars in his white coat, lean over the lectern with searching expressions, and admonish us for using psychiatric jargon or falling dumbstruck when asked how we planned to tame our patients' self-defeating side.

"How do you expect your patients to find a better and less hurtful way to live when you have no idea whatsoever about what they like to do?" he challenged (Menninger, 1938/1966,1942, 1973a, b; Menninger, Mayman, & Pruyser, 1963).

Dr. Menninger followed up with encouragement about remaining attentive and curious. His take on the value of discovering secret talents and abilities went something like this:

> It's much easier to list troubles and weaknesses than to uncover and cultivate strengths. You'll find out more than you ever imagined. You will not only be surprised by what you learn about your patient—you may learn something new from them, even about yourself.[4]

Decades before *The Queen's Gambit* television program was making headlines about a young woman's silent quest to become chess champion of the world, this patient's diagnostic conference taught me an invaluable lesson so seared into my mind that I thought I would never again miss it—of course, I have, many times. And it's always instructive when it is a "secret" talent that lands in my lap with a thud—just as it did in the case of Professor Castillo.

Given what I already knew about the professor's multiple capabilities, what had momentarily thrown me off my rocker? Why was I blind to the holistic and ever-evolving picture of her strengths? She designed, consulted on, and coordinated construction projects, had fantasies of being an architect, loved to decorate, and had hobbies of drawing and working on a loom where she used her hands. Obviously, she saw pattern and geometric shapes. Clearly, I had fumbled on a therapeutic axiom underscored throughout this entire book: there are few secrets. People want to share their truth. Look and listen for hidden treasure you may be missing. When you stumble, it's an opportunity to dig a little deeper into dynamics that may have eluded you and the patient.

Colluding or Caretaking? Patients Protect Therapists

A strength-based approach in psychotherapy isn't about dodging emotional pain, problems, or character issues but attempting to speak the language of achievement and potential also. Both clinician and patient are liable to overlook abilities for a host of psychodynamic reasons that can erupt on either side of the couch. It's the reluctance to consider, listen for, reflect upon, and even viscerally feel the strivings of the other person that needs to be analyzed. Professor Castillo's penchant for solving geometry problems blindsided me. What problem of my own might be lurking that could have subliminally signaled to her that she shouldn't be specific about this particular gift until just this moment in her analysis?

In his classic paper, "Secrets, Alliances, and Family Fictions: Some Psychoanalytic Observations," psychiatrist and psychoanalyst Theodore Jacobs (1980) describes several cases where he unconsciously colluded with his patient to avoid speaking about certain painful and embarrassing facts that they knew about him and his private life. For Jacobs, these secrets held by the patient about him included personal loss, professional setbacks, and competition with colleagues. He concludes that patients avoid bringing what they know about the therapist or the therapist's life into the open and talking about it because they fear reprisal. Should the therapist become angry, guilt ridden, or ashamed by what is revealed, the patient assumes they will be abandoned or raged against by the wounded healer. An essential attachment relationship will sever. Despair will foment. Patients seek to protect therapists when they think they will hurt our feelings or injure, another historical repetition that occurred within the early and adolescent family environment.

In retrospect, the geometry lesson between Professor Castillo and me is a case in point. I do enjoy interior decorating but have no talent whatsoever for solving geometry problems. Somewhere on the conscious-unconscious continuum, Professor Castillo—quite empathetic and insightful about the needs of her students—picked up on this about me and tried to shield me from feeling deficient in comparison to her. Jacobs explains this protective instinct:

> More often than we might be aware of, secrets of one kind or another exist between patient and analyst. Issues may arise which stir up mutual anxiety and may, consciously or otherwise, be avoided by both . . . observations that a patient has made about his analyst in areas in which he senses a narcissistic vulnerability may, as a result of a tacit understanding that develops between them, remain unspoken.
>
> (p. 40)

It's conceivable that my patient waited until she intuited that I could handle envy or shame, which, she learned in the treatment, can never be completely exorcised from the human condition. Perhaps earlier she feared what might happen if I felt in the one-down position relative to her. The event occurred as she neared the end of her analysis. By that point, there had been plenty of other opportunities to stress-test our relationship's capacity to endure her success. Just as one examines and makes space for human frailties within oneself and with one's family and friends, the patient takes note of how the analyst handles mistakes and personal shortcomings. Any propensity for idealization sifts its way out of the sandcastle.

I was able to seize the opportunity of the geometry lesson to privately mentalize and scrutinize my reactivity and raise questions in the treatment. What glimmers might Professor Castillo have about why the detail emerged when it did? Patients embark on unconscious missions to ease the burdens of their therapists, a phenomenon identified by Karlen Lyons Ruth (Macfie, Brumariu, & Lyons-Ruth, 2015; Lyons-Ruth, 2015, 2017), based on her research on how infants and children attune to the needs of a withdrawn or burdened parent. These caretaking behaviors repeat in the therapeutic relationship because the patient attempted in childhood to provide uplift, or a healing response, to their overwhelmed, traumatized, or needful primary caregivers. An unconscious secret alliance brewed.

Professor Castillo had, up to this point in her treatment, remained relatively stoic about her upbringing despite being placed in the position of caregiver for her younger siblings. She was a natural self-starter who read early and learned on her own. The professor's overworked immigrant parents provided the basics for their children but appeared unattuned to psychological needs for support and empathy. Throughout the analysis, I struggled with countertransference anger at the parents' self-preoccupation, despite being aware of the realistic cultural, financial, and time limitations they faced.

Now I began to wonder whether Professor Castillo's parents were also unconsciously competitive with their children, who they assumed would have an easier life and more opportunity than they had had. I brought this hypothesis to my patient's attention previously to see where her ideas and fantasies might take us. Not until this encounter, when I embodied in the countertransference what might have transpired long ago between her and her parents, did the dilemma about success come fully alive in the treatment. I had unconsciously taken the position of objects in the patient's inner world and identified with them, playing out what Heinrich Racker (1957) defined as a complementary countertransference reaction.

I view what occurred as an interpersonal entanglement of our non-conscious relational systems. In Professor Castillo's world, I had come to assume the position in the transference of an early attachment figure— probably both mother and father at different times in her childhood. As noted, each parent was beleaguered with work that left them with limited emotional reserves. It nevertheless boggled my mind throughout Professor Castillo's analysis that neither parent registered the dimensions of their daughter's intelligence and urged her to cultivate it.

Most caregivers do not consciously mean to do harm. In fact, every individual has their role to play in solving internal prohibitions that thwart achievement and success. As we have seen, problems are multifactorial and multifaceted in origin; psychic reality and internal conflicts about claiming talent and ability must never be given short shrift. When the interweaving of their history and unconscious fantasies is sorted through, patients usually become less fearful about owning their part of the situation—such as acknowledging their competencies and their struggle to bring them to fruition.

It's part of the therapist's task to keep in mind that we may unwittingly be getting in the way of the patient's full access to their unique gifts and taking their rightful place in the generational life cycle. They fear becoming who they are because we fear seeing who we are. The physical signs of aging constitute one visible clue that the sand in the hourglass is depleting. The timepiece will be inverted. Few gladly cede power and beauty to the next generation, even beloved progeny, a fact described by writers of myth and fairy tales ages before psychology emphasized the normative generational life cycle. Cultural stories offer another vantage point from which to appraise that ever-lurking portent, keeping talents and abilities seemingly invisible and entombed: mortality itself.

The Fairest of Them All: A Lesson for Elders from a Fairy Tale

To understand why children may unconsciously hide talents and keep abilities secret, we turn our attention to the darker side of human nature. Whether Grimm's fairy tales to contemporary children's fiction, literature reminds us that not everyone is on the child's side when it comes to championing growth and development. Likely you won't have to think long before rekindling painful childhood memories of being undercut or thwarted. Perhaps a decent, attentive family member or favorite adult whom you once adored unwittingly stole your aspirational thunder. A moment of freshly recalled teasing—maybe about falling down in high heels or showing who kicks the soccer ball farthest—can quickly spoil your good mood.

A child must endure the adult's propensity to hold on to the exulted position of authority inadvertently or deliberately, thwarting the youngster's strivings. To use characterizations from well-known fairy tales, malicious kings and queens may go so far as attempting to steal a child's birthright. Those royal evildoers set out to keep their power position—and frequently their youthful vigor—by robbing life from the underling. Their greed or envy defies the next steps in the generational life cycle that ultimately lead to the succession of the old by the young.

The fairy tale "Snow White" is a case in point.[5]

For years, the "mirror on the wall" assures Snow White's stepmother, queen of the realm, that she is the "fairest of them all"—until one day tides change. It's the mirror's function to offer honest reflection and feedback, usually in rhyme. When the Queen brings her question about her beauty once more to the mirror for reassurance, it must be truthful and declares, "Queen, you are full fair, 'tis true, But Snow White fairer is than you" (Brothers Grimm, 1812/1945, p. 163).

So begins the narrative arc of the story that leads Snow White through harrowing circumstances as the object of her stepmother's relentless pursuit to remain eternally beautiful, youthful, in charge, and alluring. Ultimately, with the help of seven dwarfs and the intervention of a prince, Snow White prevails. The child reader identifies with the protagonist's quest for individuation and selfhood and is reassured by the story: a time will come when she too succeeds her mother, who will hopefully be more charitable than the wicked stepmother.

Another, less-conscious concern has ensured the tale's universality and adaptability—it does not escape the child's unconscious, either: "Growing up must be pretty important and threatening if I have to flee for my life to do it!" The incontrovertible conflict between remaining a child forever and taking risks incumbent in individuating—and all that is attained and lost in the process—is also conveyed.

Normal human tension between generations is articulated and somewhat ameliorated by the moral of this tale. The implicit requirement for the stepmother figure is to realize she must relinquish certain assets, like beauty, as she grows older. So the adult woman reading the story to the child is getting an important message too. She still has much in her portfolio to offer, but the younger generation is gaining ground. It's clear in the story that while the queen may no longer be the most beautiful woman in the land, she is still attractive, smart, and lovable if only she could face life's natural transitions. Because she is unable to access other affirming attributes, she falters and "envy and pride like ill weeds grew higher in her heart every day until she (had) no peace day or night" (p. 163).

Then another important secret unfolds. To save her own life, Snow White pleads with the huntsman sent to kill her. To spare her life, she makes a bargain never to return to the kingdom. He acquiesces, and she runs away into the woods where she meets the seven dwarfs, who assist her newfound appreciation of her feminine wiles and keenness for self-preservation.

These two qualities of the protagonist are metaphoric stand-ins for all endowments of the younger generation that must be shrouded from the malicious adults who would "put her to death [and sell] her heart for a token" (p. 163).

Snow White, and by inference the child reader empathizing with her plight, intuits that there is more to be played out than a shift in power dynamics with her stepmother. Far in the future, she will need to step aside for the sake of her own children. Whether the young reader is precociously psychologically minded or simply remembers the facts of the tale, she gains some mastery over future challenges from the idealized version of the older women in her life. Mother, grandmother, aunt, older sibling, favorite teacher, or psychotherapy supervisor will have their struggles wanting what she has, who she may become, and coveting anything she possesses. Envy and jealously are facts of life that must be managed in the most loving and ostensibly nurturing of relationships, but there are serious deterrents to human flourishing that must be scaled. The generational life cycle is filled with expectable conflict.

Indeed, a warning comes at the end of the Brothers Grimm version of the tale, something every woman who has reached maturity should heed. Just as the marriage between the prince and Snow White is set in stone, the wicked stepmother dresses up and attempts to come to the feast. Undone by the mirror's proclamation that "a young bride is a thousand times more fair than she," the stepmother "railed and cursed beside herself with disappointment and anger" (pp. 172–173). She falls dead after seeing Snow White, vanquished in envious rage, and melting in her "red-hot iron shoes of destructiveness."

Adult readers who pause to heed the message of this fairy tale come face to face with how much more is lost than gained by trying to remain the fairest of them all forever. Knowing when to get off center stage is a secret power of elders who squarely tackle limits imposed by time, place, circumstance, and finite opportunity. Accepting the inevitable crow's feet and dancing at the wedding is a better resolution than the wicked step-mother's choice.

It Gets Darker: The Laius Complex

Flip sexes, and the remonstration is as apt for boys and men as for girls and women—save the standard of physical beauty, which is traditionally of paramount importance for women in the impossible quest for immortality. In fact, the psychological hostilities posed by generational succession are timeless and universal, the conflict made obvious (and to some extent unconsciously ameliorated) by cross-cultural phenomena from puberty rites to codified inheritance laws.

Psychoanalyst Bruno Bettelheim was among the first to popularize an additional perspective on the traditional interpretation of the Oedipus complex in his pithy classic *Freud and Man's Soul* (1983). The foundational myth of psychoanalysis rests on Oedipus's shoulders, and Bettelheim called for some needed revision and amplification.[6]

A complicated backstory leads Oedipus to kill his biological father, King Laius, and commit incest with his biological mother, Jocasta. In fact, Oedipus is abandoned by Laius, who fears the prophesy that his own son would murder and then replace him. Laius leaves his infant son to die on a mountain, but the baby is later found by another king who adopts and raises him. As a young adult, Oedipus is mortified by the prophesy that he would kill his father and marry his mother, so he flees the kingdom. His love for these parents leads him to try to escape fate. He then unknowingly kills King Laius in a brawl, never suspecting that this king is his biological father. Thus, the oracle's prophesy is inadvertently fulfilled.

Bettelheim challenges the hackneyed psychoanalytic interpretation that every boy wants to kill his father and marry his mother—the so-called Oedipus complex. Passionate longings of children to be sole possessor of their parent, usually of the opposite sex, are observable and endearing, but murderous fantasies are unconscious, time limited, and not to be taken literally.

Embedded in the broader myth is the deleterious effect of secret keeping. Once the identity of Oedipus's true parentage comes to light, "the pernicious consequences of the Oedipal deeds disappear" (Bettelheim, 1983, p. 24). Although physically blinded, Oedipus feels deep remorse and seeks reparation. Another warning is clarified: defending oneself against secrets causes "damage to oneself and others." Consequently, "becoming aware of unconscious feelings . . . purges oneself [because] feelings subside," averting "evil consequences . . . and catastrophe" (p. 25).

When Bettelheim asks what factors may have led Oedipus's father King Laius to abandon his son, he reframes the entire myth. Infanticide and filicide were known in the ancient world where the story took shape and transformed over centuries. Then, as now, the survival of children depended on the care and benevolence of parents. Inasmuch as King Laius embodied pathological narcissism, envy, and denial of mortality, he colluded with his wife to negate and destroy normative generational succession. He abrogated his paternal role as protector and nurturer of his son in the throes of an omnipotent defense: the wish to remain in his position of privilege and to live forever.

Like my interpretation of the Snow White tale, this view of the Oedipus myth is dark and comprehensive. It reflects human ambivalence about ceding power, control, and eventually life itself to the next generation. But who can even conceive of *one's own parents* wanting to destroy them? Aren't parents, and by inference other objects of transference and dependence such as teachers and mentors, supposed to love unconditionally—the well-being of progeny a central effort of adults that gives life meaning?

Fortunately for most of us, parents and other caregivers do sacrifice, and they foster the development of self, which we are then expected to do in kind for those who follow. In essence, our purpose becomes to pass on an ethic of open acceptance of finitude and to model moderation in acquisition with the prospect that advantage will accrue down the line for those we will never know. At the same time, King Laius's predicament is entirely relatable as part of the human experience—the unattainable wish to hang on indefinitely, undiminished in strength and vitality. The open secret for living the good life conveyed in the Laius-Oedipus myth is timeless: No one gets out of this life alive. Even kings do not get to have all they want. Successors who were well tended and loved will honor your memory.

The reciprocal generational takeaway for Bettelheim starts with a recognition that "in the normal course of events the son replaces the father in society as the father grows old and the son achieves manhood" (p. 28). What we know from the legend that gave us the Oedipal complex is that the "wishes and anxieties of the child have their counterparts in the feelings of the parent toward the child" (p. 29); "the myth also warns that the longer one defends oneself against knowing these secrets, the greater the damage to oneself and others" (p. 25).

Each individual is called on to reconnect with their own "inner Laius," lest one unwittingly damage the true self of someone younger. The urge to displace a rival can be mitigated by relinquishing the need for the younger person to follow in one's footsteps. This unconscious merger is one way of magnanimously sidestepping mortality and competition; grasping the ambivalent nature of love in all human relationships and the ubiquity of painful separation is another revelation.

Clinicians who keep in mind the interwoven dynamics of psychic reality, object relations, and the actual family environment are in a better position to bear the tensions of what can never be fully known about the actual events in a person's history. They can apply the knowledge gleaned from myth and fairy tales to face the darker aspects of the human condition and, to some extent, rise above them.

"I Call It Thera-Vision"

Dr. Ayman Assad was late again. I was puzzled that my supervisee's problem persisted because I had brought the issue to his attention on several occasions. What was getting in the way of punctuality? Was the supervision simply unhelpful or had something precipitated a misalliance between us? I decided to pause and simply listen to what he had on his mind after he arrived, with only twenty minutes remaining in our scheduled session.

Dr. Assad began by turning the tables on me. He said, "I have something to ask you, Dr. Z., and it's personal. I know it's probably inappropriate. It's none of my business. You can tell me to shut up and leave."

Puzzled, I silently wondered what could be so disturbing to Dr. Assad. I told him that I would try to answer if I could. At this moment, it seemed important to depart from my usual therapeutic stance of asking what lay behind his questions. He was vulnerable. I needed to be candid.

Dr. Assad continued.

I heard from another trainee that you grew up in a medical family. Your mother a nurse, your father a family doctor. How did they feel when you chose psychiatry as a specialty. I mean . . . well, was your dad okay that you didn't do what he did? I know you have published a couple of papers. Can you tell me how that sat with them too?

I felt tickled that he was asking about my family, and I was frankly relieved that Dr. Assad's questions didn't dip into waters that were embarrassing or intrusive. So I could be direct with him.

I smiled and replied,

They were both happy with my decision. My dad has read a couple of my papers. My parents joke that they don't understand a word about psychoanalysis but are glad I am making use of their investment in my education!

I let my answer sink in. The room was still. I decided to break the silence when it seemed timely. "Now it's your turn, Ayman. It must be an important question for you to ask for reasons other than learning about my parents."

He started to tear up. I thought he was sad. Then his cheeks flushed with anger like lava about to gush from a volcano.

"Do you have any idea how lucky you are? I am so jealous. I hate this field. I can't do therapy. I know I am no good at it. It's not who I am."

Looking back now, I could have been gentler. Instead, I snipped, "Then why are you here? What's keeping you from doing what you want?"

Dr. Assad said,

My parents are both mental health professionals. They love what they do and think this program is Mecca. My therapist agrees with them too. She said I should get over some kind of competitive hang-up about having a better education than they got and move on. But it's a lot more complicated than that in my family. My father would never recover if I published an academic paper, because he's never been able to do that. He's always wanted to. No one talks about it in our family but it's in the room, so to speak. My sister is a good poet and wants to publish as well as teach.

Now I understood the chronic tardiness, at least in part. Dr. Assad did not want to come to supervision because he did not want to be a therapist or psychoanalyst. He asked me his question in hopes of glomming onto an authority figure who had been in the exact position he now found himself in and who had conceived a way out from supposedly overbearing parents. My answer disappointed and then enraged my supervisee because my personal story was not the mirror he sought. Yet like most psychotherapists, I understood the inevitable tectonic shifts that occur when speaking core truths in one's family of origin. Fault lines then must be traversed in the process of separation-individuation: the establishment of a truer sense of oneself does require facing and managing emotional pain. While I was not Dr. Assad's therapist, I believed it was essential to seize the moment as his mentor and offer a different perspective in the time remaining.

I said,

> Ayman, we all make decisions and choices that disappoint people we love, like our parents. Often, they get upset and reactive when we tell them—and it can stay that way for quite a while. It's painful for them as well as for us. But ultimately, it is your life to lead. Although your loyalty is heartfelt, it can't last forever without jeopardizing who you are. You owe it to yourself—and ultimately to your parents and the world—to be who you were meant to be.

Dr. Assad was not late for supervision again. Our discussions focused on his personal dilemma. I listened as he planned how he would tell his parents that he was leaving the field of mental health; we anticipated the initial fallout that would occur when he did. For two years, he supported himself by working in a laboratory. He went on to complete another advanced degree in the physical sciences and is now widely published. Dr. Assad never pursued further psychotherapy or analysis; he found courage to override what he experienced as his father's prohibition to write, too. He has continued to stay in touch over the years and uses the insight from his own struggle for the benefit of others. I therefore have poignant follow-up on how he weathered his father's Laius complex.

During his tenure in academia, Dr. Assad has been a supervisor to a number of master's and doctoral students. He makes a point of emboldening each one to discover their passion and pursue it.

> I keep pushing back to help my students think through if they are on their unique path. I'm direct. Completing a thesis or dissertation is challenging even if it's a project that engrosses you. They tease me that I'm doing therapy with them! I joke right back. I tell them what I do is called thera-vision!

Dr. Assad's healed identification with both parents, as well as all that was absorbed throughout his truncated career in mental health, is not lost on either of us.

While technically the Laius complex in psychoanalysis refers to murderous and incestuous impulses a father has toward a son, its application takes on a broader meaning when we extend the concept to include the complicated feelings anyone in authority has toward subordinates or their own charges (Levy, 2011; Ross, 1995). Parental ambivalence and aggression can certainly undermine a child's autonomous strivings to the point of impairment in adult well-being and personal achievement. To that point, clinical data from psychotherapeutic practice, child-parent consultation, and supervisory sessions such as Dr. Assad's continue to accumulate.

Some analysts believe that the psychoanalytic profession has paid less attention to Laius than to Oedipus because it is wrenching to confront our own hostile, sadistic, and even murderous impulses toward the next generation. We deny the incontrovertible historical and anthropological evidence of ritual sacrifice, infanticide, child abuse, corporal punishment, genital mutilation, and neglecti. The knowledge is so disturbing that it remains sequestered on the conscious-unconscious continuum despite the analyst's professional requirement to undergo personal psychoanalysis and multiple supervisions of cases.

Regardless of what a caregiver consciously conveys to a child, the child also projects onto the caregiver an ideal version of themselves while omnipotently trying to fulfill that caregiver's needs and wishes. As we have seen, "wise babies" also pick up on the subliminal messages of parents and will go to great lengths to please or help them. And even the most loving and attuned parents will, at times, struggle with their child's decisions, particularly when they pierce narcissism or imbibe dissimilar values. The list of predictable conflicts and failures of mutual attunement that can set back the process of individuation is an inherently long and nuanced one. Especially injurious to healthy aspirations and innate abilities is the foreclosure by another person who perfidiously clips another's wings.

When a new patient or student asks how long their therapy or analysis will take, I elaborate on the answer I was taught in training and is still used today: "It takes as long as it takes." Knowing that secret abilities and hidden treasures will be uncovered in the treatment and need to be nourished along the way, I now add:

> Prepare for a ride on the Tilt-a-Whirl. Nurturing a truer or fuller version of yourself—your true self—is all about hills and valleys, steep inclines, unexpected spins and reverses, and jaw-dropping curves. There are many fun and fulfilling moments along the way, not just the anxiety or dread you may anticipate right now.

The discovery of a true self is an aspirational goal, never fully achieved. The qualitative difference between starting and concluding of treatment will be felt and reflected in a more vibrant daily life. Loved ones also reap rewards from these efforts, the once-defended gifts nudged to the fore along with the capacity to embrace other interests and talents yet to be discovered after termination.

Conclusion

Individuals have talents and abilities that can emerge in psychotherapy or psychoanalysis. The patient may hide or even repudiate such gifts and attributes unless a therapist infers their strengths as well as struggles and problems. Actively pursuing unrevealed talents is a more difficult task than it appears. Overriding the generational imperative of envy, jealousy, and competition is essentially what is known as the hero's journey. In many fairy tales and myths, the protagonist is repeatedly tested for fortitude and tenacity. Implied in the quest is bequeathing one's acquired power and position to the next generation in the fullness of time.

It is sometimes surprising that gems emerge in therapy that the patient never noticed beforehand, or that they feared cultivating. These pearls of recognition indicate trust in the therapeutic relationship, out of which new seeds of mastery and resilience form. After all, pearls are nothing but layer upon layer of secretions. The once-secret talent opens for collaborative elaboration. The therapist's countertransference reactions and enactments are guideposts to any stumbling blocks encountered along the way.

As long as psychotherapy lasts, clinicians will discover patients' potential, not just their problems. When an ear is kept tuned to natural endowments that may have been shelved in the past, a previously hidden chamber opens. Directions that life might have taken will need to be mourned with the support of the therapist. Psychotherapy is a second chance at catalyzing courage to reverse course that ultimately leads to a fuller, open, more satisfying life.

Together, patient and therapist must grapple with considerable emotional pleasure and anguish. Confronting intrapsychic forces and family history that propagated the need to keep talent and abilities secreted away is a labor-intensive endeavor for both patients and therapists. It is also one characteristic that makes the practice of psychotherapy as potentially life-saving and life enhancing as any of the other healing arts.

Notes

1 I am grateful to Dr. Debra Neumann, who pointed out in a discussion of this clinical example during a writing seminar that what transpired between the patient and me was an enactment. In this context, exactment means a communication in the treatment that neither the patient nor I could fully see, own, or tolerate—her talent—until this moment, for inaccessible reasons of our own. Highly embedded with specific unconscious transference and countertransference meanings, enactment can only be appreciated retrospectively. While my intention in this chapter is demonstrating a form of secret keeping on the part of patients who fear reproach or hostility from their inner objects or external environment, Dr. Neuman's observation leads me to wonder whether such turmoil is a source of enactment that goes unrecognized in psychotherapy. As such, it behooves the therapist to wonder what might be unconsciously communicated or cocreated in the dyad because of jealously, envy, competition, or

fear of being upstaged that we should subsume under the contemporary rubric of enactment.

2 Research that documents significant change rendered by psychotherapy continues to grow rapidly. Phebe Cramer's *Protecting the self: Defense mechanisms in action* (2006) and Wilma Bucci and William Cornell's *Emotional communication and therapeutic change: Understanding psychotherapy through multiple code theory* (2021) are two recent publications that expand on modes of change in ego function and quality of life as described in the earlier Menninger Clinic studies.

3 Personal communication, Peter Novotny, MD, September 1981.

4 Seminars with Dr. Karl A. Menninger, 1978, 1981, 1982.

5 For an especially graphic cinematic rendering of the Snow White dynamic, see the 2012 film *Snow White and the Huntsman*. The wicked stepmother queen Ravenna (Charlise Theron) attempts to become immortal by sucking youth from young maidens. She demands her minions successively bring attractive girls to her and then proceeds to inhale their vitality, fixating on them as they shrivel into decrepit eyesores. Theron's character grows visibly youthful and more stunning every time her chosen victim is maliciously aspirated into her body. The audience is held captive as witness to the evil inspiration. The visual stunts and photographic effects of this live-action movie are terrifying but depict the embodied fantasy of a female rival's refusal to gracefully age. Contrast that with the classic Disney cartoon version (1938), where the stepmother's oral rage and need to destroy are kept largely off-screen as Snow White frolics with the seven dwarfs and eventually collapses after choking on a poison apple—until the prince saves her. Camouflaged by a whimsical musical score and the virtuous attitude of the gentle main characters, sins of envy, greed, sadism, and the desire to rob life from Snow White are made deceptively palatable to innocent eyes. No doubt the unconscious message still comes through because this film version remains immensely popular after nearly one hundred years. Apparently, children have a need to be reassured that their natural strivings toward maturity and having a family of their own will ultimately win out over the ambivalent and destructive urges they intuitively sense from even their most loving and generous of attachment figures—who make sure they see the film but will ultimately be replaced by them in the life cycle.

6 Bettelheim was summarizing the original research of anthropologist and psychoanalyst George Devereux (1953), whom he does not cite in his short, highly readable text. Devereux's scholarship ferrets out more details of the traumatic family lineage of the mythic King Laius that led to his sadistic actions toward his son Oedipus. By placing the Oedipus myth in expanded cultural and historical context, this paper raised serious questions about the organizing stories and symbols that psychoanalysts use to base our assumptions, make clinical interventions, expand existing theories, and understand psychosexual development. Multidisciplinary efforts like Devereux's may demonstrate, as he concluded, that "the task of psycho-analytic research will never be finished" (1953, p. 139), but curiously only a few analysts have followed his lead by taking Laius as a central figure needing psychoanalytic scrutiny and applying these insights to clinical cases. Given the ubiquity and depth of psychic pain and conflict derived from impasses in generational succession, including within the field of psychoanalysis itself beginning with Freud, failure to confront and analyze the Laius complex in adults is a serious scotoma—and a kept secret—within the psychoanalytic profession but for a few noteworthy exceptions (see Levy, 2011; Ross, 1982, 1983, 1995, 2007).

Epilogue

Three months after beginning psychotherapy, Marshall still hadn't uttered one word.

With each stonewalled encounter, my frustration and embarrassment escalated. Simple questions, banal comments about the weather, and attempts to suggest an emotion or trauma that might underpin such deep silence—they all met with rebuke. Usually, Marshall just closed his eyes and pretended to go to sleep.

My supervisor, Dr. Richardson, sensed discouragement and sought to soothe escalating anxiety about the psychotherapy process. "I have the feeling that it's going to take a long of time for Marshall to let you in," he advised. "If you do hang in there, he will make some progress. You will, too. Be patient. Don't lose hope."

* * *

Well-meaning advice and suggestions from experts were useful over the next three years, but no dramatic change occurred. Those meetings with Marshall played out as a kind of game in my mind, and I wonder, decades after the fact, how many other clinical novices seek a magic solution when unable to engage a reluctant patient. Instead of "visiting professor rounds," colloquy should perhaps be called by its rightful name: "Stump the Authority."

During that difficult period, supervision sessions became pivotal place markers, giving me the stability to let time unfold. They made it easier to "hang in there" and "be patient" because they helped abate my feelings of inadequacy while still proceeding at the patient's pace. Supervision imparted essential lessons about the growth factors that underpin psychotherapy, while imperceptibility fostering change.

Gradually, the thirty-five-year-old Marine veteran Marshall started to speak—tentatively—and took a part-time job on the grounds as custodian. It was a good day when he shouted from the corridor: "Yo, Doc! It's me, Marshall!" He even took the stick of gum I offered.

* * *

DOI: 10.4324/9781003471578-9

Balm for a therapist arrives serendipitously.

During an evening seminar on child psychotherapy, a senior clinician shared that he once treated a young boy who neither played nor spoke. This therapist had griped about the patient over dinner with his wife, who asked, "Well, do you talk to him?" Abashedly, the senior clinician owned that he rarely said much.

His wife allegedly shot back, "How do you think babies learn to speak? We mutter, we sing, we murmur to them. Little ones especially perk up when you say their name in a story. Talk to the boy!"

Following that evening class, I began to speak to Marshall differently. I hummed as we strolled across the VA grounds. I chortled whenever thorns in the rose garden put a run in my pantyhose. I chatted about marshals in the army and navy, in the generic and the specific: US marshals on airplanes. Marshal Wyatt Earp. Marshaling our strength to make one more trip around the parking lot in the Kansas snow before time was up. One afternoon, he trusted me to reveal the hideout of a litter of feral kittens he fed. I named each one after a psychoanalytic pioneer I knew from the literature. Marshall nodded affirmatively at the choices, even though I was sure he didn't know the players: Harry, Clara, Otto, Anna, and, my favorite, Siggy, their mischievous ginger tabby papa.

* * *

Over seven years, a thaw did occur with Marshall. First a trickle of spare sentences, it began to flow and eventually cascaded into him talking about wildlife he saw on our rounds. We continued to walk the hospital grounds and greet people on the pathways. One day, we paused by the fountain. Marshall turned and stared sternly into my eyes. With an eerie baritone I had never heard before, he said, "I know who you were in a past life."

Across the span of a few sessions, he revealed a delusion that I, a teenager in the thirteenth century, was raped and murdered by a group of mercenaries, only to be reborn in the fifteenth century as a prostitute. "I will keep this information to myself until I can find a way to redeem us both," he decided.

* * *

From that point on, Marshall's internal world unfolded over months, paved with the violence, greed, hatred, perversity, and split-off wishes for reparation that I was reading about in psychoanalytic training. Evenings, excited by the breakthrough, I would search through articles and texts that could help me craft an interpretation the next time he brought his panoramic delusional world to our sessions.

A mere minute into our next meeting, the opportunity arrived. He began, "Apollo is coming back next year and then . . . ."

Brimming with interventions from the texts, I jumped full force into the pool of my reflections—until I hit a wall. I tried to pull threads together, but my garbled phrases exposed that I was stuck in a jumble of conflicting concepts. I missed the mark. I knew it.

"Marshall," I said, "I am not making any sense today, not even to myself. I'm sorry."

"That's OK, Dr. Z. I understand. You've studied lots of ideas. You need to practice them. What's important for me is that you listen."

Now I was the one rendered speechless.

* * *

This treatment would never be considered successful by typical markers. Still, as the attending psychiatrist at the mental health clinic put it, Marshall created "an unusual life for himself—but still, a life." He maintained a part-time custodian job in town and volunteered at a local animal shelter, making regular financial contributions to it. The highlight of his year was hosting a Thanksgiving celebration at a local diner for fifteen to twenty of his buddies who were also lonely veterans without family. He always invited me to join, but I respectfully declined. By the time taps blew for Marshall, we had worked together for more than twenty-three years.

* * *

"I have no idea why Marshall's treatment is on my mind today," I told a colleague over cappuccino.

> He's been dead for well over twenty years. I believe I mentioned that he came by bus to Portland to meet a couple of times in person after I moved here, and we still chatted from time to time on the phone.

"Yes, you have. I remember Marshall," she said, taking a bite of a marionberry scone.

"I still have his Purple Heart in a cupboard in my office," I confessed.

At the start of a therapy session, Marshall had taken the medal out of a sack and dropped it on my side table. He said, "I am leaving it here or throwing it in the trash." Ten years into the treatment, I knew when to leave well enough alone, or so I thought. I persisted in trying to bring up the deposit but to no avail.

A couple months later, he set the record straight. "You know the Purple Heart is really for you, don't you? I'm never taking it back. And you earned it," he said.

"What in the world do you mean?" I asked him. "You know I can't keep this in my office forever. Let's keep talking about it. There must be someone you know who . . . ."

He interrupted me in midsentence, which was unusual. "Remember the night you killed the wasp. You're brave!"

My colleague broke into the story I was telling: "What in the world was he talking about? A fantasy or a dream?"

Marshall had called in crisis. I told him I could talk but first had to extinguish a wasp that had landed in the dining room and was frightening everybody. After that deed was done, I returned to chat for a few moments and noticed he had calmed down.

"He knew you could handle stingers!" she giggled.

"He never let me forget the wasp story, either."

"I'm not surprised. Patients remember moments like those. They're human. And show vulnerability."

"What exactly do you mean?" I asked, savoring another sip to stymie tears. I still missed him.

"I think you know exactly what I mean. Patients understand that we, too, get wounded in the trenches. It takes courage to enter their world. It's been hidden in such deep silence for so long," she said.

"Working with Marshall was an education."

"I hear that," she said.

We always remain their students, but patients study us the whole time. Their vault opens gradually.

"Better hold on to that medal then," she advised.

"And do what with it?"

"Tell the story."

References

Abassi, A. (2014). "Have you heard?" Revelations regarding the analyst. In *The rupture of serenity: External intrusions and psychoanalytic technique* (pp. 47–68). London: Karnac.

Abassi, A. (2018). The analyst's bodily sensations as important information in clinical work. *Psychoanalytic Inquiry, 38*, 530–540.

Abend, S. (1982). Serious illness in the analyst: Countertransference considerations. *Journal of the American Psychoanalytic Association, 30*, 365–379.

Abraham, N. (1975). Notes on the phantom: A complement to Freud's metapsychology. In T. Rand (Ed. & Trans.), *The shell and the kernel: Renewals of psychoanalysis* (Vol. 1, pp. 171–176). Chicago, IL: University of Chicago Press.

Abraham, N., & Torok, M. (1972). Mourning or melancholia: Introjection versus incorporation. In T. Rand (Ed. & Trans.), *The shell and the kernel: Renewals of psychoanalysis* (Vol. 1, pp. 125–138). Chicago, IL: University of Chicago Press.

Abraham, N., & Torok, M. (1973). Self-to-self affliction: Notes of a conversation on "psychosomatics." In T. Rand (Ed. & Trans.), *The shell and the kernel: Renewals of psychoanalysis* (Vol. 1, pp. 162–164). Chicago, IL: University of Chicago Press.

Abraham, N., & Torok, M. (1975). "The lost object–me": Notes on endocryptic identification. In T. Rand (Ed. & Trans.), *The shell and the kernel: Renewals of psychoanalysis* (Vol. 1, pp. 139–156). Chicago, IL: University of Chicago Press.

Abraham, N., & Torok, M. (1994). *The shell and the kernel: Renewals of psychoanalysis* (Ed. & Trans. T. Rand, Vol. 1). Chicago, IL: University of Chicago Press.

Adler, G. (1979). The psychotherapy of schizophrenia: Semrad's contributions to current psychoanalytic concepts. *Schizophrenia Bulletin, 5*, 130–157.

Akhtar, S. (1992). Tethers, orbits, and invisible fences: Clinical, developmental, sociocultural, and technical aspects of optimal distance. In S. Kramer & S. Akhtar (Eds.), *When the body speaks: Psychological meanings in kinetic clues* (pp. 21–58). Northvale, NJ: Jason Aronson.

Akhtar, S. (2000). Mental pain and the cultural ointment. *International Journal of Psychoanalysis, 81*, 229–243.

Akhtar, S. (2001). From mental pain through manic defense to mourning. In S. Akhtar (Ed.), *Three faces of mourning: Melancholia, manic defense, and moving on* (pp. 95–114). Northvale, NJ: Jason Aronson.

Allen, J. G. (2002). Coping with the catch-22s of depression: A guide for educating patients. *Bulletin of the Menninger Clinic, 66*, 103–144.

Allen, J. G. (2013). *Restoring mentalizing in attachment relationships: Treating trauma with plain old therapy*. Washington, DC: American Psychiatric Press.

Allen, J. G. (2022). *Trusting in psychotherapy*. Washington, DC: American Psychiatric Press.

Amir, D. (2008). Naming the nonexistent: Melancholia as mourning over a possible object. *Psychoanalytic Review, 95*, 1–15.

Amir, D. (2012). The inner witness. *International Journal of Psychoanalysis, 93*, 879–896.

Anderegg, D. (2005). "You're not a Freudian, are you?" Secret identities in the lives of working clinicians. *American Journal of Psychoanalysis, 65*, 333–339.

Appelbaum, S. (1977). *The anatomy of change: A Menninger Foundation report on testing the effects of psychotherapy*. New York: Plenum.

Appelbaum, S. (1978). Pathways to change in psychotherapy. *Bulletin of the Menninger Clinic, 41*, 511–521.

Appelbaum, S. (1981). *Effecting change in psychotherapy*. New York: Jason Aronson.

Apprey, M. (1998). Staging and transforming historical grievances: From a culture of memory to a reconstructable future. *Psychoanalysis, Culture and Society, 3*, 81–90.

Apprey, M. (1999). Reinventing the self in the face of transgenerational hatred in the African American Community. *Journal of Applied Psychoanalytic Studies, 1*, 131–143.

Apprey, M. (2006). Differences and the awakening of wounds in international psychoanalysis. *The Psychoanalytic Quarterly, 75*, 73–93.

Apprey, M. (2014a). "Containing the uncontainable": The return of the phantom and its reconfiguration in ethnonational conflict and resolution. *American Journal of Psychoanalysis, 74*, 162–175.

Apprey, M. (2014b). A pluperfect errand: A turbulent return to beginnings in the transgenerational transmission of destructive aggression. *Free Associations, 15*, 6–29.

Armstrong, K. (2004). *The spiral staircase: My climb out of darkness*. New York: Knopf.

Attig, T. (2004). Disenfranchised grief revisited: Discounting hope and love. *OMEGA–Journal of Death and Dying, 49*, 197–215.

Auchincloss, E. L., & Samberg, E. (2012). *Psychoanalytic terms and concepts*. New Haven, CT: American Psychoanalytic Association/Yale University Press.

Avery, N. C. (1982). Family secrets. *Psychoanalytic Review, 69*, 47–486.

Balsam, R. H. (2015). Eyes, ears, lips, fingertips, secrets: Dora, psychoanalysis, and the body. *Psychoanalytic Review, 102*, 33–58.

Barratt, B. B. (2013). Free-associating with the bodymind. *International Forum of Psychoanalysis, 22*, 161–172.

Barrett, L. F. (2020). *7 & ½ lessons about the brain*. Boston, MA: Houghton, Mifflin, Harcourt.

Barrett, L. F., & Finlay, B. L. (2018). Concepts, goals and the control of survival-related behaviors. *Current Opinion in Behavioral Sciences, 24*, 172–179.

Barrett, L. F., & Quigley, K. S. (2021). Interception: The secret ingredient, *Cerebrum*. cer-06–21.

Basseches, H. (1988). Transgenerational haunting: Interview with Maurice Apprey. *The American Psychoanalyst, 36*, 15, 32.

Bernfeld, S. (1941). The facts of observation in psychoanalysis. *International Review of Psychoanalysis, 12*, 342–351.

Bettelheim, B. (1983). *Freud and man's soul*. New York: Knopf.

Bion, W. R. (1962). *Learning from experience*. London: Heinemann.

Bion, W. R. (1970). *Attention and interpretation*. London: Heinemann.

Bion, W. R. (1975). *Bion's Brazilian lectures II*. Rio de Janeiro: Imago Editora.

Blos, P. (1962). *On adolescence: A psychoanalytic interpretation*. New York: Simon & Schuster.

Blos, P. (1979). *The adolescent passage: Developmental issues*. New York: International Universities Press.

Blum, A., Goldberg, P., & Levin, M. (2023). *Here I am alive: The spirit of music in psychoanalysis*. New York: Columbia University Press.

Bok, S. (1978). *Lying: Moral choice in public and private life*. New York: Vintage.

Bok, S. (1983). *Secrets: On the ethics of concealment and revelation*. New York: Vintage.

Bonhoeffer, D. (1965/1978). What is meant by "telling the truth"? In S. Bok (Ed.), *Lying: Moral choice in public and private life* (pp. 282–286). New York: Vintage.

Borgogno, F. (2022). *One life heals another: Beginnings, maturity, outcomes of a vocation*. New York: International Psychoanalytic Books.

Bowlby, J. (1979). On knowing what you are not supposed to know and feeling what you are not supposed to feel. *Canadian Journal of Psychiatry, 241*, 403–408.

Brandchaft, B. (1985). Resistance and defense: An intersubjective view. *Progress in Self Psychology, 1*, 88–96.

Brandchaft, B. (1988). A case of intractable depression. *Progress in Self Psychology, 4*, 133–154.

Brandchaft, B. (2001). Obsessional disorders: A developmental systems perspective. *Psychoanalytic Inquiry, 21*, 253 288.

Brandchaft, B. (2002). Reflections on the intersubjective foundations of the sense of self: Commentary on paper by Steven Stern. *Psychoanalytic Dialogues, 12*, 727–745.

Brandchaft, B. (2007). Systems of pathological accommodation and change in analysis. *Psychoanalytic Psychology, 24*, 667–687.

Brandchaft, B., Doctors, S., & Sorter, D. (2010). *Toward an emancipatory psychoanalysis: Brandchaft's intersubjective vision*. London: Routledge.

Brockman, R. (2023). Safety: From the Paris morgue to oxytocin. *Journal of Psychoanalysis and Psychodynamic Psychiatry, 50*, 585–602.

Brown, L. J. (2012). Bion's discovery of alpha function: Thinking under fire on the battlefield and consulting room. *International Journal of Psychoanalysis, 93*, 1191–1214.

Bucci, W. (1997). *Psychoanalysis and cognitive science: A multiple code theory*. New York: Guilford Press.

Bucci, W. (2008). New perspectives on the multiple code theory: The role of bodily experience in emotional organization. In F. S. Anderson (Ed.), *Bodies in treatment: The unspoken dimension* (pp. 51–77). Hillsdale, NJ: Analytic Press.

Bucci, W. (2011a). The interplay of subsymbolic and symbolic processes in psychoanalytic treatment: It takes two to tango—but who knows the steps, who's the leader? The choreography of psychoanalytic interchange. *Psychoanalytic Dialogues, 21,* 45–54.

Bucci, W. (2011b). The role of subjectivity and intersubjectivity in the reconstruction of dissociated schemas: Converging perspectives from psychoanalysis, cognitive science, and affective neuroscience. *Psychoanalytic Psychology, 28,* 247–266.

Bucci, W. (2018). Emotional communication in the case of Antonio. *Psychoanalytic Inquiry, 38,* 518–529.

Bucci, W., & Cornell, W. (Eds.) (2021). *Emotional communication and therapeutic change: Understanding psychotherapy through multiple code theory.* New York: Routledge.

Carignan, L. (1999). The secret: A study of perverse transference. *International Journal of Psychoanalysis, 80,* 909–928.

Copeland, L. (2020). *The lost family: How DNA testing is upending who we are.* New York: Abrams Press.

Cozolino, L. (2017). *The neuroscience of psychotherapy: Healing the social brain.* 3rd ed. New York: W. W. Norton.

Cramer, P. (2006). *Protecting the self: Defense mechanisms in action.* New York: Guilford Press.

Critcher, C. R., & Ferguson, M. J. (2014). The cost of keeping it hidden: Decomposing concealment reveals what makes it depleting. *Journal of Experimental Psychology: General, 143,* 721–735.

Devereux, G. (1953). Why Oedipus killed Laius: A note on the complementary Oedipus complex in Greek drama. *International Journal of Psychoanalysis, 34,* 132–141.

Doka, K. J. (1999). Disenfranchised grief. *Bereavement Care, 18,* 37–39. doi: 10.1080/02682629908657467

Doka, K. J. (Ed.) (2002). *Disenfranchised grief. New directions, challenges, and strategies for practice.* Champagne, IL: Research Press.

Druss, R. G. (1995). *The psychology of illness in sickness and in health.* Washington, DC: American Psychiatric Press.

Druss, R. G. (2000). *Listening to patients: Relearning the art of healing in psychotherapy.* London: Oxford University Press.

Durban, J. (2016). Shadows, ghosts, and chimeras: On some early modes of handling psycho-genetic heritage. In A. Harris, M. Kalb, & S. Klebanoff (Eds.), *Ghosts in the consulting room: Echoes of trauma in psychoanalysis* (pp. 76–96). New York: Routledge.

Eagle, M. N. (2018). *Core concepts in classical psychoanalysis: Clinical, research evidence and conceptual critiques.* New York: Routledge.

Eagleman, D. (2020). *Livewired: The inside story of the ever-changing brain.* New York: Vintage.

Ellenberger, H. F. (1966). The pathogenic secret and its therapeutics. *Journal of the History of Behavioral Sciences*, 2, 29–42.

Ellenberger, H. F. (1970). *The discovery of the unconscious: The history and evolution of dynamic psychiatry*. New York: Basic Books.

Feldman, M. (2016). Transgenerational trauma and witnessing in analyst and analysand. In A. Harris, M. Kalb, & S. Klebanoff (Eds.), *Ghosts in the consulting room: Echoes of trauma in psychoanalysis* (pp. 52–75). New York: Routledge.

Field, N. (1988). Listening with the body: An exploration in the countertransference. *British Journal of Psychotherapy*, 5, 512–522.

Frankfeldt, V. (2019). Incongruent feeling states. *Psychoanalytic Inquiry*, 3–4, 268–275.

Franks, L. (2007). *My father's secret war. A memoir* New York: Hyperion.

Freud, S. (1895). The psychotherapy of hysteria. In J. Strachey (Ed. & Trans.), *The standard edition of the complete psychological works of Sigmund Freud* (Vol. 2, pp. 225–305). London: Hogarth Press.

Freud, S. (1905a). Fragments of an analysis of a case of hysteria. In J. Strachey (Ed. & Trans.), *The standard edition of the complete psychological works of Sigmund Freud* (Vol. 7, pp. 3–122). London: Hogarth Press.

Freud, S. (1905b). On psychotherapy. In J. Strachey (Ed. & Trans.), *The standard edition of the complete psychological works of Sigmund Freud* (Vol. 7, pp. 257–268). London: Hogarth Press.

Freud, S. (1913). On beginning the treatment. In J. Strachey (Ed. & Trans.), *The standard edition of the complete psychological works of Sigmund Freud* (Vol. 12, pp. 121–144). London: Hogarth Press.

Freud, S. (1915/1917). Mourning and melancholia. In J. Strachey (Ed. & Trans.), *The standard edition of the complete psychological works of Sigmund Freud* (Vol. 14, pp. 243–258). London: Hogarth Press.

Freud, S. (1919). The uncanny. In J. Strachey (Ed. & Trans.), *The standard edition of the complete psychological works of Sigmund Freud* (Vol. 17, pp. 217–252). London: Hogarth Press.

Freud, S. (1921). Group psychology and the analysis of the ego. In J. Strachey (Ed. & Trans.), *The standard edition of the complete psychological works of Sigmund Freud* (Vol. 16, pp. 67–144). London: Hogarth Press.

Freud, S. (1940). An outline of psycho-analysis. In J. Strachey (Ed. & Trans.), *The standard edition of the complete psychological works of Sigmund Freud* (Vol. 23, pp. 144–207). London: Hogarth Press.

Fromm-Reichman, F. (1960). *Principles of intensive psychotherapy*. Chicago, IL: University of Chicago Press.

Gabbard, G. (1989). On "doing nothing" in psychoanalytic treatment of the refractory borderline patient. *International Journal of Psychoanalysis*, 70, 527–534.

Gallese, V. (2006). Mirror neurons and intentional attunement: Commentary on olds. *Journal of the American Psychoanalytic Association*, 54, 47–57.

Gallese, V. (2011). Embodied simulation theory: Imagination and narrative. *Neuropsychoanalysis*, 13, 196–200.

Ginot, E. (1997). The analyst's use of self, self-disclosure, and enhanced integration. *Psychoanalytic Psychology*, 14, 365–381.

Ginot, E. (2007). Intersubjectivity and neuroscience: Understanding enactments and their significance within emerging paradigms. *Psychoanalytic Psychology*, 24, 317–332.

Ginot, E. (2009). The empathic power of enactments: The link between neuropsychological processes and an expanded definition of empathy. *Psychoanalytic Psychology*, 26, 290–309.

Ginot, E. (2015). *The neuropsychology of the unconscious: Integrating brain and mind in psychotherapy*. New York: W. W. Norton.

Giuliano, R. J., Karns, C. M., Bell, T. A., Peterson, S., Skowron, E. A., Neville, H. J., & Pakulak, N. E. (2018). Parasympathetic and sympathetic activity are associated with individual differences in neural indices of selective attention in adults. *Psychophysiology*, 55, 8. doi: 10.1111/psyp.13079.

Goldberg, A. (1999). *Being of two minds: The vertical split in psychoanalysis and psychotherapy*. Hillsdale, NJ: Analytic Press.

Goldberg, N. (1986). *Writing down the bones: Freeing the writer within*. Boulder, CO: Shambhala Publications.

Grand, S. (2000). *The reproduction of evil: A clinical and cultural perspective*. Hillsdale, NJ: Analytic Press.

Grand, S. (2003). Lies and body cruelties in the analytic hour. *Psychoanalytic Dialogues*, 13, 471–500.

Grand, S. (2016). Vaginal ghosts: Memorializing the disappeared. In A. Harris, M. Kalb, & S. Klebanoff (Eds.), *Ghosts in the consulting room: Echoes of trauma in psychoanalysis* (pp. 97–112). New York: Routledge.

Grimm, J., & Grimm, W. (1812/1945). Snow-White and the seven drafts. In E. V. Lucas, L. Crane, & M. Edwardes (Trans.), *Grimm's Fairy Tales* (pp. 162–173). New York: Grosset & Dunlap.

Gross, A. (1951). The secret. *Bulletin of the Menninger Clinic*, 15, 37–44.

Grossman, L. (Host) (2023, May 28). Technique is character rationalized (No. 135) [audio podcast episode]. In *Off the Couch: An IPA Podcast*. International Psychological Association. https://ipaoffthecouch.org/2023/05/28/episode-135-technique-is-character-rationalized-with-lee-grossman-md-oakland-ca/

Grotstein, J. (1997). Why Oedipus and not Christ? A psychoanalytic inquiry into innocence, human sacrifice, and the sacred, part II: The numinous and spiritual dimension as a metapsychological perspective. *American Journal of Psychoanalysis*, 57, 317–335.

Grotstein, J. (2000). *Who is the dreamer who dreams the dream? A study of psychoanalytic presences*. Hillsdale, NJ: Analytic Press.

Grotstein, J. (2007). *A beam of intense darkness: Wilfred Bion's legacy to psychoanalysis*. London: Karnac.

Gubb, K. (2014). Craving interpretation: A case of somatic countertransference. *British Journal of Psychotherapy*, 30, 51–67.

Gut, E. (1989). *Productive and unproductive depression*. New York: Basic Books.

Hagman, G. (1995). Mourning: A review and reconsideration. *International Journal of Psychoanalysis*, 76, 909–925.

Hagman, G. (1996). The role of the other in mourning. *Psychoanalytic Quarterly*, 65, 327–352.

Halpert, E. (2000). On lying and the lie of a toddler. *Psychoanalytic Quarterly*, 69, 659–675.

Hamilton, R., Vohs, K. D., Sellier, A.-L., & Meyvis, T. (2011). Being of two minds: Switching mindsets exhausts self-regulatory resources. *Organizational Behavior and Human Decision Processes*, 115, 13–14. doi: 10.1016/j.obhdp.2010.11.005

Harris, A., Kalb, M., & Klebanoff, S. (Eds.) (2016). *Ghosts in the consulting room: Echoes of trauma in psychoanalysis*. New York: Routledge.

Harris, A., & Sinsheimer, K. (2008). The analyst's vulnerability: Preserving and fine-tuning analytic bodies. In F. S. Anderson (Ed.), *Bodies in treatment: The unspoken dimension* (pp. 255–273). New York: Analytic Press.

Heatherton, T. F., & Wagner, D. D. (2011). Cognitive neuroscience of self-regulation failure. *Trends in Cognitive Science*, 15, 132–139. doi: 10.1016/j.tics.2010.12.005

Hoyt, M. F. (1978). Secrets in psychotherapy: Theoretical and practical considerations. *International Review of Psychoanalysis*, 5, 231–241.

Hoyt, M. F. (1980). Secrets in psychotherapy. *International Review of Psychoanalysis*, 7, 407–408.

Imber-Black, E. (1998). *The secret life of families*. New York: Bantam Books.

Jacobs, T. J. (1980). Secrets, alliances, and family fictions: Some psychoanalytic observations. *Journal of the American Psychoanalytic Association*, 28, 21–42.

Jacobs, T. J. (1987). Notes on the unknowable: Analytic secrets and the transference neurosis. *Psychoanalytic Inq*uiry, 7, 485–509.

Jaffe, E. (2006). The science behind secrets. *APS Observer*. https://www.psychologicalscience.org/observer/the-science-behind-secrets.

James, K., & Engelhardt, L. (2012). The effects of handwriting experience on functional brain development in pre-literate children. *Trends in Neuroscience and Education*, 1, 32–42.

Jaques, E. (1965). Death and the mid-life crisis. *International Journal of Psychoanalysis*, 46, 502–514.

Kandel, E. R., Koester, J. D., Mack, S. H., & Siegelbaum, S. A. (Eds.) (2022). *Principles of neural science* (6th ed.). New York: McGraw-Hill.

Kernberg, O., Burstein, E., Coyne, L., Appelbaum, A., Horwitz, L., & Voth, H. (1972). Psychotherapy and psychoanalysis: Final report of the Menninger Foundation's Psychotherapy Research Project. *Bulletin of the Menninger Clinic, 36*, 3–274.

Khan, M. (1974). *The privacy of the self*. London: Hogarth Press.

Khan, M. (1983). *Hidden selves: Between theory and practice in psychoanalysis*. London: Karnac.

King, S., & Chizmar, R. (2017). *Gwendy's button box*. New York: Gallery Books.

Klein, M. (1940). Mourning and its relation to manic-depressive states. *International Journal of Psychoanalysis*, 21, 125–153.

Knapp, C. (1996). *Drinking: A love story*. New York: Dial Press.

Knoblauch, S. H. (2000). *The musical edge of therapeutic dialogue*. Hillsdale, NJ: Analytic Press.

Knoblauch, S. H. (2005). Body rhythms and the unconscious: Toward an expanding of clinical attention. *Psychoanalytic Dialogues*, 15, 807–827.

Knoblauch, S. H. (2008). Attention to the analyst's subjectivity: From Kohut to now.... How are we doing? *International Journal of Psychoanalytic Self Psychology*, *3*, 237–239.

Knoblauch, S. H. (2011). Contextualizing attunement within the polyrhythmic weave: The psychoanalytic samba. *Psychoanalytic Dialogues*, *15*, 203–209.

Knoblauch, S. H. (2017). The fluidity of emotions and clinical vulnerability: A field of rhythmic tensions. *Psychoanalytic Perspectives*, *14*, 283–308.

Knoblauch, S. H. (2018). Attention and narration to micro-moment registrations of embodied dialogue in the clinical interaction: How are we doing? *Psychoanalytic Inquiry*, *38*, 502–510.

Krestan, J., & Bepko, C. (1993). On lies, secrets, and silence: The multiple levels of denial in addictive families. In E. Imber-Black (Ed.), *Secrets in families and family therapy* (pp. 141–159). New York: W. W. Norton.

Krupp, G. (1965). Identification as a defence against anxiety in coping with loss. *International Journal of Psychoanalysis*, *46*, 303–314.

Kulish, N. (2002). Female sexuality: The pleasure of secrets and the secrets of pleasure. *Psychoanalytic Study of the Child*, *57*, 151–179.

Lane, D. M., & Pearson, D. A. (1982). The development of selective attention. *Merrill-Palmer Quarterly*, *28*, 317–337.

Lane, J. D., & Wegner, D. M. (1995). The cognitive consequences of secrecy. *Journal of Personality and Social Psychology*, *69*, 237–253.

Lapid, M. I., Chen, Y., Rummans, T. A., McAlpine, D. E., & Zerbe, K. J. (2013). Eating disorders in later life: A clinical review. *Clinical Geriatrics*, *21*. Advance online publication.

Lathrop, D. (2017). Disenfranchised grief and physician burnout. *Annals of Family Medicine*, *15*, 375–378.

Lelio, S. (Director & Writer), & Maza, G. (Writer) (2017). *A fantastic woman* [film]. Fabula.

Leuzinger-Bohleber, M. (2008). Biographical truths and their clinical consequences: Understanding "embodied memories" in a third psychoanalysis with a traumatized patient recovered from severe poliomyelitis. *International Journal of Psychoanalysis*, *89*, 1165–1187.

Leuzinger-Bohleber, M. (2015a). *Finding the body in the mind: Embodied memories, trauma, and depression*. London: Karnac.

Leuzinger-Bohleber, M. (2015b). Working with severely traumatized, chronically depressed analysands. *International Journal of Psychoanalysis*, *96*, 611–636.

Leuzinger-Bohleber, M. (2021). Psychoanalysis and community: Migration, flight, and trauma. *Psychoanalytic Dialogues*, *31*, 522–523.

Leuzinger-Bohleber, M., Kallenbach, L., & Schoett, M. J. (2016). Pluralistic approaches to the study of process and outcome in psychoanalysis. The LAC depression study: A case in point. *Psychoanalytic Psychotherapy*, *30*, 4–22.

Leuzinger-Bohleber, M., Solms, M. E., & Arnold, S. E. (Eds.) (2020). *Outcome research and the future of psychoanalysis: Clinicians and researchers in dialogue*. New York: Routledge.

Levenson, E. A. (2005a). *The ambiguity of change*. New York: Analytic Books.

Levenson, E. A. (2005b). *The fallacy of understanding*. New York: Analytic Books. (Original work published 1972).

Levy, I. (2011). The Laius complex: From myth to psychoanalysis. *International Forum of Psychoanalysis*, *20*, 222–228.

Little, M. I. (1981). *Transference neurosis and transference psychosis*. New York: Jason Aronson.

Little, M. I. (1990). *Psychotic anxieties and containment: A personal record of an analysis with Winnicott*. Northvale, NJ: Jason Aronson.

Loewald, H. W. (1960). On the therapeutic action of psychoanalysis. *International Journal of Psychoanalysis*, *41*, 16–33.

Loewenberg, P. (2017). Freud as an existential humanistic psychotherapist: The case of Margarethe. *Journal of the American Psychoanalytic Association*, *65*, 665–672.

Lyons-Ruth, K. (2015). Dissociation and the parent–infant dialogue. A longitudinal perspective from attachment research. *Attachment: New Directions in Relational Psychoanalysis and Psychotherapy*, *9*, 253–276.

Lyons-Ruth, K. (2017). Revisiting the idealizing transference: "Needful things" and the Faustian bargain. *Psychoanalysis, Self, and Context*, *12*, 197–210.

Macfie, J., Brumariu, L. E., & Lyons-Ruth, K. (2015). Parent-child role confusion. A critical review of an emerging concept. *Developmental Review*, *36*, 34–57.

Malawista, K. (2021a, May 26). A passageway out of pandemic loss: How to put grief and trauma into a faraway nearby. *Boston Globe*.

Malawista, K. (2021b). *The things they carry project*. https://www.thingstheycarryproject.org.

Maranges, H. F., & Baumeister, R. F. (2016). Self-control and ego depletion. In K. D. Vohs & R. F. Baumeister (Eds.), *Handbook of self-regulation* (3rd ed., pp. 42–61). New York: Guilford Press.

Margolis, G. (1966). Secrecy and identity. *International Journal of Psychoanalysis*, *47*, 517–522.

Margolis, G. (1974). The psychology of keeping secrets. *International Review of Psychoanalysis*, *1*, 291–296.

Markman, H. C. (2020). Embodied attunement and participation. *Journal of the American Psychoanalytic Association*, *68*, 807–834.

Markman, H. C. (2022). *Creative engagement in clinical practice*. New York: Routledge.

Marks-Tarlow, T. (2011). Merging and emerging: A nonlinear portrait of intersubjectivity during psychoanalysis. *Psychoanalytic Dialogues*, *21*, 110–127.

Marks-Tarlow, T. (2014). Context is everything! [Review of the book *Psychoanalytic complexity: Clinical attitudes for therapeutic change*, by William Coburn]. *International Journal of Psychoanalytic Self Psychology*, *9*, 392–396.

Marks-Tarlow, T. (2015). Commentary on dynamical systems theory: Theory and practical applications. *Psychoanalytic Dialogues*, *25*, 131–135.

Maroda, K. J. (2022). *The analyst's vulnerability: Impact on theory and practice*. New York: Routledge.

Masur, C. (2001). Can women mourn their mothers? In S. Akhtar (Ed.), *Three faces of mourning: Melancholia, manic defense, and moving on* (pp. 33–46). Northvale, NJ: Aronson.

Mazower, M. (2017). *What you do not tell: A father's past and the journey home*. New York: Other Press.

Meares, R. (1988). The secret, lies, and the paranoid process. *Contemporary Psychoanalysis, 24,* 650–666.

Menninger, K. (1938/1966). *Man against himself.* New York: Harcourt, Brace, and World.

Menninger, K. (1942). *Love against hate.* New York: Harcourt, Brace, and World.

Menninger, K. (1973a). *Whatever became of sin?* New York: Hawthorn.

Menninger, K. (1973b). *Sparks.* L. Freeman (Ed.). New York: Crowell.

Menninger, K. A., Mayman, M., & Pruyser, P. (1963). *The vital balance: The life process in mental health and illness.* New York: Viking Press.

Mueller, P. A., & Oppenheimer, D. M. (2014). The pen is mightier than the keyboard: Advantages of longhand over laptop note taking. *Psychological Science, 25,* 1159–1168. doi: 10.1177/0956797614524581

Mullahy, P. (1970). *The beginnings of modern American psychiatry: The ideas of Harry Stack Sullivan.* Boston, MA: Houghton Mifflin.

Murphy, K. (2019). *You're not listening: What you're missing and why it matters.* New York: Celadon Books.

Novick, K. K., & Novick, J. (2010). *Emotional muscle.* Xlibris.

Ogden, T. H. (2004a). An introduction to the reading of Bion. *International Journal of Psychoanalysis, 85,* 285–300.

Ogden, T. H. (2004b). On holding and containing, being and dreaming. *International Journal of Psychoanalysis, 85,* 1349–1364.

Ogden, T. H. (2007). Elements of analytic style: Bion's clinical seminars. *International Journal of Psychoanalysis, 88,* 1185–1200.

Orgad, Y. (2014). On family secrets and -K. *International Journal of Psychoanalysis, 95,* 771–789.

Panksepp, J. (2009). Brain emotional systems and qualities of mental life: From animal models of affect to implications for psychotherapeutics. In D. Fosha, D. J. Siegel, & M. F. Solomon (Eds.), *The healing power of emotion: Affective neuroscience, development, and clinical practice* (pp. 1–26). New York: W. W. Norton.

Panksepp, J., & Biven, L. (2012). *The archaeology of mind: Neuroevolutionary origins of human emotions.* New York: W. W. Norton.

Peebles, M. J. (1983). Handling psychiatric emergency: or, Keeping one's diagnostic wits in a crisis. *Bulletin of the Menninger Clinic, 47,* 453–471.

Peebles, M. J. (2008). Trauma-related disorders and dissociation. In M. R. Nash & A. J. Barnier (Eds.), *The Oxford handbook of hypnosis: Theory, research, and practice* (pp. 647–679). Oxford: Oxford University Press.

Peebles, M. J. (2018). Harm in hypnosis: Three understanding from psychoanalysis can help. *American Journal of Clinical Hypnosis, 60,* 239–261.

Peebles, M. J. (2022). *When psychotherapy feels stuck.* New York: Routledge.

Pennebaker, J. W. (1989). Confession, inhibition, and disease. *Advances in Experimental Social Psychology, 22,* 211–244.

Pennebaker, J. W. (1993). Putting stress into words: Health, linguistic, and therapeutic implications. *Behavioral Research and Therapy, 31,* 539–548.

Pennebaker, J. W., & Beal, S. K. (1986). Confronting a traumatic event: Toward an understanding of inhibition and disease. *Journal of Abnormal Psychology, 95,* 274–281.

Pennebaker, J. W., & Chung, C. (2007). Expressive writing, emotional upheavals, and health. In H. S. Friedman & R. C. Silver (Eds.), *Foundations of health psychology* (pp. 263–284). New York: Oxford.

Pennebaker, J. W., & Smyth, J. M. (2016). *Opening up by writing it down: How expressive writing improves health and eases emotional pain* (3rd ed.). New York: Guilford Press.

Pennebaker, J. W., & Susman, J. R. (1988). Disclosure of trauma and psychosomatic processes. *Social Science and Medicine, 26*, 327–332.

Peskin, J., & Ardino, V. (2003). Representing the mental world in children's social behavior: Playing hide-and-seek and keeping a secret. *Social Development, 12*, 496–512. doi: 10.1111/1467–9507.00245

Peterfreund, E. (1971). *Information, systems, and psychoanalysis.* New York: International University Press.

Peterfreund, E. (1972). On information-processing models of mental phenomena: A response to Lawrence Friedman's critical review of "Information, systems, and psychoanalysis" by Emanuel Peterfreund. *International Journal of Psychoanalysis, 54*, 351–357.

Peterfreund, E. (1980). On information and systems models for psychoanalysis. *International Review of Psychoanalysis, 7*, 327–345.

Peterfreund, E. (1990). On the distinction between clinical process and clinical content theories. *Psychoanalytic Psychology, 7*, 1–12.

Petrucelli, J. (2010). Things that go bump in the night: Secrets after dark. In J. Petrucelli (Ed.), *Knowing, not-knowing & sort-of-knowing: Psychoanalysis and the experience of uncertainty* (pp. 135–149). London: Karnac.

Pizer, A. (2016). Do I have to tell my patients I'm blind? *Psychoanalytic Perspectives, 13*, 214–229.

Pizer, S. A. (2009). Inside out: The state of the analyst and the state of the patient. *Psychoanalytic Dialogues, 19*, 49–62.

Plude, D. J., Enns, J. T., & Brodeur, D. (1994). The development of selective attention: A life-span overview. *Acta Psychologica, 86*, 227–272.

Polley, S. (Director & Writer) (2012). *The stories we tell* [film]. National Film Board of Canada.

Polley, S. (Director & Writer) (2022). *Women talking* [film]. Adapted from M. Toews (2018), *Women talking.* New York: Knopf.

Polley, S. (2022). *Run toward the danger: Confrontations with a body of memory.* New York: Penguin.

Power, A. (2016). *Forced endings in psychotherapy and psychoanalysis: Attachment and loss in retirement.* New York: Routledge.

Powers, R. G. (1998). Introduction. In D. Moynihan (Ed.), *Secrecy: The American experience* (pp. 1–58). New Haven, CT: Yale University Press.

Quinodoz, D. (2009). *Growing old: A journey of self-discovery.* New York: Routledge.

Racker, H. (1957). The meaning and uses of countertransference. *Psychoanalytic Quarterly, 26*, 303–357.

Rand, N. T. (1994a). New perspectives in metapsychology: Cryptic mourning and secret love. In T. Rand (Ed. & Trans.) *The shell and the kernel: Renewals of psychoanalysis* (Vol. 1, pp. 99–106). Chicago, IL: University of Chicago Press.

Rand, N. T. (1994b). Secrets and posterity: The theory of the transgenerational phantom. In T. Rand (Ed. & Trans.) *The shell and the kernel: Renewals of psychoanalysis* (Vol. 1, pp. 165–169). Chicago, IL: University of Chicago Press.

Raskin, E. (1992). *Family secrets and the psychoanalysis of narrative.* Princeton, NJ: Princeton University Press.

Raskin, E. (2008). *Unspeakable secrets.* Albany: State University of New York.

Reiner, A. (2012). *Bion and being.* London: Karnac.

Reiner, A. (Ed.) (2017). *Of things invisible to mortal sight: Celebrating the work of James Grotstein.* London: Karnac.

Richman, S. (2009). Secrets and mystifications. Finding meaning through memoir. *Psychoanalytic Perspectives, 6,* 67–75.

Richman, S. (2012). *A wolf in the attic: The legacy of a hidden child of the Holocaust.* New York: Routledge.

Roberto, L. G. (1993). Eating disorders and family secrets. In E. Imber-Black (Ed.), *Secrets in families and family therapy* (pp. 160–177). New York: W. W. Norton.

Rosen, V. H. (1955). Reconstruction of a traumatic childhood event in a case of derealization. *Journal of the American Psychoanalytic Association, 3,* 211–221.

Ross, J. M. (1982). Oedipus revisited: Laius and the "Laius complex." *Psychoanalytic Study of the Child, 37,* 169–200.

Ross, J. M. (1983). Father to the child: Psychoanalytic reflections. *Psychoanalytic Review, 70,* 301–320.

Ross, J. M. (1995). King Oedipus and the postmodern psychoanalyst. *Journal of the American Psychoanalytic Association, 43,* 959–961.

Ross, J. M. (2007). Trauma and abuse in the case of Little Hans: A contemporary perspective. *Journal of the American Psychoanalytic Association, 55,* 779–797.

Roth, P. (2007). Melancholia, mourning, and the countertransference. In L. G. Fiorini, T. Bokanowski, & S. Lewkowicz (Eds.), *On Freud's "Mourning and melancholia"* (pp. 37–56). London: International Psychological Association.

Samberg, E. (2004). Resistance: How do we think of it in the twenty-first century? *Journal of the American Psychoanalytic Association, 52,* 243–253.

Sandler, J. (1976). Countertransference and role responsiveness. *International Review of Psychoanalysis, 3,* 43–47.

Sayette, M. A., & Creswell, K. G. (2016). Self-regulatory failure and addition. In K. D. Vohs & R. F. Baumeister (Eds.), *Handbook of self-regulation* (3rd ed., pp. 571–589). New York: Guilford.

Schlesinger, H. J. (2005). *Endings and beginnings. On terminating psychotherapy and psychoanalysis.* Hillsdale, NJ: The Analytic Press.

Shabad, P. (1987). Fixation and the road not taken. *Psychoanalytic Psychology, 4,* 187–205.

Shabad, P. (1993). Repetition and incomplete mourning. *Psychoanalytic Psychology, 10,* 61–75.

Shapiro, Y., & Marks-Tarlow, T. (2021). Varieties of clinical intuition: Explicit, implicit, and nonlocal neurodynamics. *Psychoanalytic Dialogues, 31,* 262–281.

Slavin, J. H., & Rahmani, M. (2016). Those 45 minutes changed my life: The meeting of Sigmund Freud and Margarethe Lutz. *Psychoanalytic Perspectives, 13,* 291–293.

Slepian, M. L., Chun, J. S., & Mason, M. F. (2017). The experience of secrecy. *Journal of Personality and Social Psychology, 113*, 1–33.

Slepian, M. L., & Greenaway, K. H. (2018). The benefits and burdens of keeping others' secrets. *Journal of Experimental Social Psychology, 78*, 220–232.

Slepian, M. L., Kirby, J. N., & Kalokerinos, E. K. (2020). Shame, guilt, and secrets on the mind. *Emotion, 20*, 323–328.

Sletvold, J. (2011). The reading of emotional expression: Wilhelm Reich and the history of embodied analysis. *Psychoanalytic Dialogues, 21*, 453–467.

Sletvold, J. (2012). Training analysts to work with unconscious embodied expressions: Theoretical underpinnings and practical guidelines. *Psychoanalytic Dialogues, 22*, 410–429.

Sletvold, J. (2014). *The embodied analyst: From Freud to Reich to relationality.* New York: Routledge.

Sletvold, J. (2016). The analyst's body: A relational perspective from the body. *Psychoanalytic Perspectives, 13*, 186–200.

Sletvold, J., & Brothers, D. (2021). Talking bodies: A new vision of psychoanalysis. *Psychoanalytic Inquiry, 42*, 289–302.

Stolorow, R. D., & Brandchaft, B. (1987). Developmental failure and psychic conflict. *Psychoanalytic Psychology, 4*, 241–253.

Sullivan, H. S. (1954). *The psychiatric interview.* H. S. Perry & M. L. Gawel (Eds.). New York: W. W. Norton.

Symington, J., & Symington, N. (1996). *The clinical thinking of Wilfred Bion.* London: Routledge.

Taber, S. M. (2012). *Born under an assumed name: The memoir of a Cold War spy's daughter.* Dulles, VA: Potomac Books.

Thompson, C. M. (1964). *Interpersonal psychoanalysis: The selected papers of Clara M. Thompson.* New York: Basic Books.

Tillman, J. (2016). The intergenerational transmission of suicide: Moral injury and the mysterious object in the work of Walker Percy. *Journal of the American Psychoanalytic Association, 64*, 541–568.

Torok, M. (1968). The illness of mourning and the fantasy of the exquisite corpse. In T. Rand (Ed. & Trans.), *The shell and the kernel: Renewals of psychoanalysis* (Vol. 1, pp. 107–124). Chicago, IL: University of Chicago Press.

Van Gerven, P. M. V., & Guerreiro, M. J. S. (2016). Selective attention and sensory modality in aging: Curses and blessings. *Frontiers in Human Neuroscience, 10*, Article 147. doi: 10.3389/fnhum.2016.00147

Vivona, J. M. (2009a). Embodied language in neuroscience and psychoanalysis. *Journal of the American Psychoanalytic Association, 57*, 1327–1215.

Vivona, J. M. (2009b). Response to commentaries. *Journal of the American Psychoanalytic Association, 57*, 569–573.

Volkan, V. D. (1981). *Linking objects and linking phenomena: A study of the forms, symptoms, metapsychology, and therapy of complicated mourning.* New York: International Universities Press.

Volkan, V. D. (1984). Complicated mourning. In C. Kligerman (Ed), *Annual of Chicago institute of psychoanalysis* (pp. 323–348). Chicago, IL: University of Chicago Press.

Volkan, V. D. (1999). Psychoanalysis and diplomacy, part III: Potentials for and obstacles against collaboration. *Journal of Applied Psychoanalytic Studies, 1,* 305–318.

Volkan, V. D. (2007). Not letting go from individual perennial mourners to societies with entitlement ideologies. In L. G. Fiorini, T. Bokanowski, & S. Lewkowicz (Eds.), *On Freud's "Mourning and melancholia"* (pp. 90–109). London: International Psychological Association.

Volkan, V. D. (2013). Large-group psychology in its own right: Large -group identity and peace making. *International Journal of Applied Psychoanalytic Studies, 10,* 210–246.

Volkan, V. D. (2017). Psychoanalytic thoughts on the European refugee crisis and the other. *Psychoanalytic Review, 104,* 661–685.

Wachtel, P. L. (2023). *Making room for the disavowed: Reclaiming the self in psychotherapy.* New York: Guilford Press.

Wagner, D. D., & Heatherton, T. F. (2013). Self-regulatory depletion increases emotional reactivity in the amygdala. *Social Cognitive and Affective Neuroscience, 8,* 410–417. doi: 10.1093/scan/nss082

Wagner, D. D., & Heatherton, T. F. (2015). Self-regulation and its failure: The seven deadly threats to self-regulation. In M. Mikulincer, P. R. Shaver, E. Borgida, & J. A. Bargh (Eds.), *APA handbook of personality and social psychology: Attitudes and social cognition* (Vol. 1, pp. 805–842). Washington, DC: American Psychological Association. doi: 10.1037/14341-026

Waller, J. (1992). *The bridges of Madison County.* New York: Warner.

Wallerstein, R. (1986). *Forty-two lives in treatment: A study of psychoanalysis and psychotherapy.* New York: Guilford.

Wallerstein, R. (1992). Follow up in psychoanalysis: What happens to treatment gains. *Journal of the American Psychoanalytic Association, 40,* 665–690.

Warsaw, S. C. (1996). The loss of my father in adolescence: Its impact on my work as a psychoanalyst. In B. Gerson (Ed.), *The therapist as a person* (pp. 207–222). Hillsdale, NJ: Analytic Press.

Warsaw, S. C. (2018). Review of the book *Healing after parent loss in childhood and adolescence. Therapeutic interventions and theoretical consideration,* by P. Cohen, K. M. Sossin, & R. Ruth (Eds.), with a foreword by N. McWilliams (2014). New York: Rowman and Littlefield *Psychoanalytic Psychology, 34,* 350–252.

Wegner, D. M. (1989). *White bears and other unwanted thoughts: Suppression, obsession, and the psychology of mental control.* New York: Penguin Press.

Wegner, D. M. (2011). Setting free the bears: Escape from thought suppression. *American Psychologist, 66,* 671–680.

Wegner, D. M., Schneider, D. J., Carter, S. R., & White, T. L. (1987). Paradoxical effects of thought suppression. *Journal of Personality and Social Psychology, 53,* 5–13.

Wegner, D. M., & Schneider, D. J. (2003). The white bear story. *Psychological Inquiry, 14,* 326–329.

Wegner, D. M., & Zanakos, S. (1994). Chronic thought suppression. *Journal of Personality, 62,* 615–640.

Weir, K. (2020). Exposing the hidden world of secrets. *American Psychological Association Monitor, 51,* 74.

Wilson, M. (2018). The analyst as listening-accompanist: Desire in Bion and Lacan. *Psychoanalytic Quarterly, 87,* 237–264.

Wollan, M. (2017, July 17). How to read palms. *New York Times Magazine.*

Wooldrige, T. (Ed.) (2018). *Psychoanalytic treatment of eating disorders: When words fail and bodies speak.* New York: Routledge.

Worrall, C. (2015). Commentary on "Craving interpretation: A case of somatic countertransference," by K. Gubb. *Journal of Analytical Psychology, 60,* 575–577.

Zerbe, K. (1993a). *The body betrayed: Women, eating disorders, and treatment.* Washington, DC: American Psychiatric Press. (Published in paperback, Carlsbad, CA: Gurze Books, 1995).

Zerbe, K. (1993b). Selves that starve and suffocate: The continuum of eating disorders and dissociative phenomena. *Bulletin of the Menninger Clinic, 57,* 319–327.

Zerbe, K. (1993c). Whose body is it anyway? Understanding and treating psychosomatic aspects of eating disorders. *Bulletin of the Menninger Clinic, 57,* 161–177.

Zerbe, K. (1995). Integrating feminist and psychodynamic principals in the treatment of an eating disorder patient: Implications for using countertransference responses. *Bulletin of the Menninger Clinic, 59,* 160–176.

Zerbe, K. (1998). Knowable secrets. Transference and countertransference manifestation in eating disorder patients. In W. Vandereyken & P. J. Beaumont (Eds.), *Treating eating disorders* (pp. 30–55). London: Athlone Press.

Zerbe, K. (2001). The crucial role of psychodynamic understanding in the treatment of eating disorders. *Psychiatric Clinics of North America, 24,* 305–313.

Zerbe, K. (2007). Psychodynamic management of eating disorders. In J. Yager & P. Powers (Eds.), *Clinical manual of eating disorders* (pp. 307–334). Washington, DC: American Psychiatric Press.

Zerbe, K. (2008). *Integrated treatment of eating disorders: Beyond the body betrayed.* New York: W. W. Norton.

Zerbe, K. (2016). Psychodynamic issues in the treatment of binge eating disorder: Working with shame, secrets, no-entry, and false body defenses. *Clinical Social Work Journal, 44,* 8–17. doi: 10.1007/s10615-015-0559-9

Zerbe, K. (2019). The secret life of secrets: Deleterious psychosomatic effects on patient and analyst. *Journal of the American Psychoanalytic Association, 67,* 185–214. doi: 10.1177%2F0003065119826624

Zerbe, K. (2020). Pandemic fatigue: Facing the body's inexorable demands in the time of COVID–19. *Journal of the American Psychoanalytic Association, 68,* 475–478.

Zerbe, K. (2022a). Aches, pains, rumbles, and stumbles: Applying somatic countertransference and body reactivity in clinical work and teaching. *Psychoanalytic Review, 109,* 167–193.

Zerbe, K. (2022b). The analyst's self-care: Further reflections on cultivating resilience and the essential role of the body-mind relationship in clinical practice. *Psychodynamic Psychiatry, 50,* 603–621.

Zerbe, K., Becker, A. E., & Yager, J. (2002). Eating disorders: Update. *Psychiatric Update, 22*, 1–10

Zerbe, K., & Bradley, K. (2018). Bring me your hungers: Omnipotence, mourning, and the inexorable limits of time in the psychodynamic treatment of eating disorders. *Psychoanalytic Review, 105*, 363–395. doi: 10.1521/prev.2018.105.4.363

Zerbe, K., & Satir, D. A. (2016). Psychodynamic improvement in eating disorders: Welcoming ignored, unspoken, and neglected concerns in the patient to foster development and recovery. *International Journal of Child and Adolescent Psychotherapy, 15*, 259–277. doi: 10.1080/15551024.2016.1107408. Also published in Tom Wooldridge (Ed.) (2019). *Psychoanalytic treatment of the eating disorders: When words fail and bodies speak* (pp. 17–42). London: Routledge.

Index

Note: Page numbers followed by "n" denote endnotes.

Abassi, A. 135–136
Abend, S. 134–135
Abraham, N. 88–90
Anderegg, D.: "Secret Identities in the Lives of Working Clinicians" 132
anxiety-packed queries 51
Apprey, M. 87
Armstrong, K.: *The Spiral Staircase: My Climb Out of Darkness* 32n2
authoritarian psyche 20
autonomic nervous system 49

Balsam, R. H. 108
Barratt, L. F. 107, 119–120
Bernfeld, S. 28; "The Facts of Observation in Psychoanalysis" 27
Bettelheim, B. 161–162, 167n6; *Freud and Man's Soul* 160
Bion, W. R. 145, 148n1
body budget 119–123
Bok, E. S. 21, 131
bonds of intimacy 42
Born under an Assumed Name: The Memoir of a Cold War Spy's Daughter (Taber) 95–98
Bowlby, J. 41, 43, 49, 54
brain-based mechanisms 4, 73, 122
Brandchaft, B. 53, 54
The Bridges of Madison County (Johnson) 64
Bucci, W. 76n1, 110
burden of secrecy 33–37, 44–45, 50–53; complicate grieving 39–41; Landon's psychotherapy 53–55; moral injury 56–58; spiral of

healing 55–56; weights on the body 46–50; weights on the mind 41–44

Carignan, L. 138; "autonomy and identity" 137
Carrigan, L. 144
Chizmar, R.: *Gwendy's Button Box* 48
classical psychoanalysis, fundamental rule of 16
clinicians cultivate modes of concealment 127
cognitive neuroscience 110, 122
cognitive psychology 7, 43, 63, 66, 107
complicated ethical decision-making process 7
complicated ethics of concealment 125–127, 129–132, 147–148; containment and transformation 138–140; safe-deposit box 140–145; secret wars in the mind 145–147; therapist's camouflage 127–129; therapist's secret identities 132–138
"conscious–unconscious continuum" 4, 98, 105, 133, 156, 165
containment and transformation 138–140
contemporary biology 49
contemporary cognitive psychology 66
contemporary psychoanalysts 38
contemporary psychodynamic practice 148n1
contemporary psychotherapeutic technique 109
contemporary psychotherapy research 93–95

Copeland, L.: *The Lost Family: How DNA Testing Is Upending Who We Are* 76n1
cortical maps 119
Critcher, C. 65

depression 36, 41, 50, 51
Devereux, G. 167n6
dichotic listening 45
disenfranchised grief 64, 70–71, 75
distinct emotional systems 49
double lives 6, 68–70, 133
DPV and LAC research groups 95, 100n5
Druss, R. 96

Earp, M. W. 169
Eliot, T. S.: "Ash Wednesday" 32n2; *Four Quartets* 32n2
Ellenberger, H. F. 24, 25
emotional catharsis mode 108
emotional exhaustion 37, 50, 58, 71
emotional processing, in subsymbolic formats 110
espionage agents 28, 127, 145
ethical decision-making 7, 145, 147
ethics *see* complicated ethics of concealment
excessive stress 49
excretory release 108
explicit permission 43, 58

Fairbairn, W. R. D. 100n3
"false secret" 23
family ghosts 84
A Fantastic Woman (Chilean film) 70–71
Ferguson, M. J. 65
Frankfeldt, V. 69–70
Franks, L. 146, 148; *My Father's Secret War: A Memoir* 127, 145
Franks, T. 145–147
Freud and Man's Soul (Bettelheim) 160
Freud, S. 10, 21, 28, 31n1, 37, 38, 108, 123n1, 132
Fromm-Reichman, F. 34

Galatzer-Levy, R. 139
Gates, H. L. 76n1
gender differences 12
generational life cycle 158, 160
glucocorticoid receptor regulatory feedback mechanisms 49

goals of psychotherapy 85–86, 94–95
Goldberg, N.: *Writing Down the Bones* 71
Grand, S. 137–138, 144
grief and grieving 5, 38–41, 55, 56, 61, 63, 64, 69–72, 75, 76, 88, 90
Gross, A. 108
Grossman, L. 32n1
Growing Old: A Journey of Self-Discovery (Quinodoz) 67
Gwendy's Button Box (King and Chizmar) 48

"healthy denial" 96
heimlich 21
helical model 32n2
hidden talents and abilities 149–152; fairy tale 158–160; Laius complex 160–162; patients protect therapists 155–158; remember to ask 153–155; thera-vision 162–165; treasures 152–153
Holocaust 6, 52, 87, 88, 92, 95, 146
homeostasis 48, 99
hospitalization 56
Hoyt, M. 16
hypothalamic-pituitary-adrenal (HPA) axis 48, 49

identification 38–40, 56, 76n1, 132, 137, 164
"the illness of mourning" 87–89, 91
intensive psychotherapy and psychoanalysis 93
intergenerational ghosts 80, 86, 99
interiority 24, 108
intrapsychic: crypts 88, 91, 99; ghosts 96; phantoms 83

Jacobs, T. 136–137; "Secrets, Alliances, and Family Fictions: Some Psychoanalytic Observations" 156
Jacques, E. 52; "a doer" 51
Johnson, F. 64–65, 73; *The Bridges of Madison County* 64

Kincaid, R. 64, 65
King, S.: *Gwendy's Button Box* 48
Klein, M. 56
Knapp, C. 69–70; *Drinking: A Love Story* 68
Krupp, G. 39
Kulish, N. 109

Laius complex in psychoanalysis 160–162, 164, 167n6
latent cues 152
lens of contemporary psychotherapy research 93–95
Leuzinger-Bohleber, M. 94, 95, 100n5; "plurality of methods" 93
Levenson, E. 34
linchpin 5, 67
Litella, E. 75
Little, M. I. 139, 148n1
Loewald, H. 85
longer-term psychotherapy 24

Mahler, M. 39
Malawista, K. 72
masquerades 138
memory suppression 41
Menninger, K. 154, 155
metabolic dysfunction 49
mind-body dissociation 96
mirror neuron system 112–114, 120
moral injury, psychodynamics of suicide 56–58
Morin, S. 114–120
mourning process 36–40, 55, 56, 63, 67, 87, 93, 99
multigenerational: hauntings 87, 96; phantoms 80, 83, 86–88, 99
multiple code theory 76n2
Murphy, K.: *You're Not Listening: What You're Missing and Why It Matters* 32n1
My Father's Secret War: A Memoir (Franks) 127, 145

Neumann, D. 166n1
neuromodulatory systems 118
neurophysiological processes 4
neuropsychology 112
neuroscience 7, 8, 49, 77, 107, 112; cognitive neuroscience 110, 122
nonconscious relational systems 157
nonverbal cues 18, 62
normative defense 96

Oedipal phase of development 39
Oedipus complex 160–162, 165
Orgad, Y. 147

parasympathetic system 49
parentified child 42, 57, 66, 129, 152, 162, 165

parietal cortex 118
Pascal's aphorism 141
paternal suicide 56
pathogenic secret 24–28, 31
pathological accommodation 43, 53, 54
patients protect therapists 155–158
Peebles, M. J. 100n1
Pennebaker, J. 73
personal identifiers 132
Peterfreund, E. 45
Petrucelli, J. 133, 134, 144
pharmacotherapy 94
physical and emotional burden, of secret keeping 6, 63, 66
physical illness 5, 33, 89, 107
physical relief for secret 24, 31
physiologic system 109
Pizer, A. 135
Pizer, S. 135
"plurality of methods," by Leuzinger-Bohleber 93
Polley, S.: *Run toward the Danger: Confrontations with a Body of Memory* 123n2; *Stories We Tell* 110–112
Power, A. 108
power of secrets 11–18; challenge of secret keeping 28–31; essential etymological essence in the word 20–21; pathogenic secrets 24–28; souvenir 22–24; spiral staircase 18–20
Powers, R. G. 20
precise defensive strategy 105
protective camouflage 148
protective psychological function 58, 89
psychiatry 8, 11, 12, 24, 97, 162; illness 39, 50, 54, 87; jargon 154
psychic: crypts 87, 90–93; enclaves 87; warts 47–48
psychic pain: layers of 99; ubiquity and depth of 167n6
psychoanalysis/psychoanalytic 12, 43, 64, 87, 152, 166; Laius complex in 160–162, 164, 167n6; theory 83–84; training 8, 115, 169
psychodynamics: authors 132; consultation 28; practice 15; psychotherapy 27, 43, 64, 83, 87, 102, 152; of suicide 56; therapy 40
"psychological vault or crypt" 89
psychology/psychological process 108, 158; cognitive psychology

7, 43, 63, 65, 107; contemporary cognitive psychology 66; distress 5; hostilities 160; neuropsychology 112; phantoms and ghost 82–83, 99; and physical well-being 95; real-life psychology 44; relief for secret 24, 31, 34; research 23, 44; turbulence 98
psychopathology 23
psychosis 35, 97
psychotherapy/psychotherapeutic process 4, 10, 16, 18, 71, 72, 77n2, 78, 104, 122, 127, 166, 168; confidence in 19; elderly patients in 67; "emancipatory" 53; goal of 85–86; intensive 93; Landon's psychotherapy 53–55; longer-term 24; origins of 5; practice of 12, 145, 165; psychodynamic 27, 43, 64, 83, 87, 102, 152; self-discovery in 19; self-reflective process of 34; spiral staircase during 18–20; strength-based approach in 155; training 130

The Queen's Gambit television program 155
Quinodoz, D. 70; *Growing Old: A Journey of Self-Discovery* 67

Racker, H. 157
Radner, G.: *Saturday Night Live* 75
randomized controlled trials 93–94
real-life psychology 44
relief 6, 25, 72, 85, 105, 113, 117; psychological/physical relief 24, 31, 34
Richman, S. 52
robust positive effect 99
Roos, P. 123n1
Rosen, I. 59n1
Ruth, K. L. 157

safe-deposit box 140–145
Sandler, J. 136
Schlesinger, H. J.: *Endings and Beginning: On Terminating Psychotherapy and Psychoanalysis* 32n2
secret identities, therapists 132–138
secretion 20, 49, 166

secret keeper/secret keeping 56, 66, 71–73, 125, 127–129, 136, 144, 146; accumulated repercussions of 49; challenge of 28–31; chronic stress of 58; complex 24; convolution and layering of 8; deleterious effect of 161; depositories for 6; double lives 6, 68–70, 133; emotional and physical consequences of 68; impact of 44; in Landon's family 57; layers of 55; organizing function of 52; phenomenon of 48; physical and psychological effects of 44; power and burdens of 9; primary negative emotion associated with 46; psychological and physical effects of 62–63; residual effect of 69; secrets and 50; and secret sharing 17, 43; suicide 37, 56, 57, 69, 70, ubiquity of 7
secrets 7, 9; burden of *see* burden of secrecy; complicated ethics of concealment *see* complicated ethics of concealment; "false secret" 23; hidden talents and abilities *see* hidden talents and abilities; joyous secrets 45–46; listening to 10; pathogenic secret 24–28, 31; physical relief for 24, 31; power of *see* power of secrets; somatic countertransference *see* somatic countertransference; themes of 5; "unspeakable secrets" 5, 87, 99; wars, in the mind 145–147
self-regulatory depletion 65–67
Selman, M. 11, 16, 18
Semrad, E. 106, 107; "tour of the body" technique 102
separation-individuation process 55, 165
shame 15, 25, 27, 38, 39, 42, 46, 54, 71–73, 91, 92, 108, 130, 135–138, 142, 156
"side effects" of keeping secrets 46
single-case-study method 94
Slepian, M. 44–46, 49
Sletvold, J. 103, 105–107
"Snow White" (fairy tale) 9, 158–161, 167n5
somatic countertransference 101–103, 121–123; clinician's body's reactivity 105–107; consultation sessions

103–104; Morin, Stacy 114–120;
pleasure 107–109; reactions,
working with 109–110; role of
mirror neurons 112–114; *Stories
We Tell* 110–112; "Talk, Walk, and
Write" 120–121, 123
spiral of healing 55–56
spiral staircase, during psychotherapy
18–20
spontaneity of interaction 28
Stories We Tell (Polley) 110–112
stress-induced neural dysregulation 49
structured psychological interview 28
subsymbolic systems 110
suicide 5, 33, 36, 37, 41–43, 48, 49,
51, 56, 57, 69, 70
Sullivan, H. S. 34
"The Suzie Swanky Story" 13
symbiotic enmeshment 53
sympathetic system 49
"system of pathological
accommodation" 54

Taber, S.: *Born under an Assumed
Name: The Memoir of a Cold War
Spy's Daughter* 95–98
"Talk, Walk, and Write"
120–121, 123
therapeutic process 143, 147

therapists: camouflage 127–133, 138;
countertransference reactions and
enactments 166; patient and 166;
patients protect 155–158; secret
identities 132–138
thera-vision 162–165
Thomas, M. 60
Thompson, C. 34
Tillman, J. 56, 57
Torok, M. 88–90
"tour of the body" technique, by
Semrad 102
transgenerational: ghosts 83;
transmission of trauma 87, 93–97,
99, 100n1, 100n4

unheimlich 21
"unspeakable secrets" 5, 87, 99
unwanted ghost 82, 99

Volkan, V. 40

Walter, M. 123n1
Wegner, D. M. 44, 46, 49
White Bear story 44–45
Winnicott, D. W. 139–140, 148n1, 152
Writing Down the Bones (Goldberg) 71

Zerbe, K. 100n2, 123n3

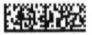